Earn CME credits while you

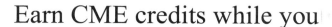

Up to 75 *AMA PRA Category 1 Credits*™ available with the MedStudy 2011 Internal Medicine Board-Style Questions & Answers

Release Date: December 1, 2010   Expiration Date: December 1, 2013

To apply for CME credit, you must complete the **Verification of Credit** form and the **Product Evaluation** found on the next pages. Then submit the completed form and evaluation, along with the $40 CME processing fee, to MedStudy.

Please note: CME credit is available **only** to the original purchaser of this product, and issuance of CME credit is subject to verification of product ownership.

To be eligible for CME credit, you must study the content in the books and submit your Verification of Credit form and Evaluation to MedStudy no later than **December 1, 2013**. (1 hour = 1 CME credit)

Continuing Medical Education

MedStudy is accredited by the Accreditation Council for Continuing Medical Education (ACCME) to provide continuing medical education for physicians.

MedStudy designates this educational activity for a maximum of 75 *AMA PRA Category 1 Credits*™. Physicians should only claim credit commensurate with the extent of their participation in the activity.

Learning Objectives

As a result of participation in this activity, learners will be able to:

- Integrate and demonstrate increased overall knowledge of Internal Medicine

- Identify and remedy areas of weakness (gaps) in knowledge and clinical competencies

- Describe the clinical manifestations and treatments of diseases encountered in Internal Medicine and effectively narrow the differential diagnosis list by utilizing the most appropriate medical studies

- Apply the competence and confidence gained through participation in this activity to both a successful Board exam-taking experience and daily practice

Target Audience / Method of Participation

Participants in this educational activity are those physicians seeking to expand and reinforce their knowledge and clinical competencies in Internal Medicine, focusing one's learning on subjects that are directly relevant to clinical scenarios that will be encountered on the ABIM Certification or Recertification Board exam, as well as in the practice setting. The content of this CME activity is intended to help learners assess their own key knowledge and clinical competencies with evidence-based standards of care, which are reflected on the Board exams. Use the question-answer content as a self-study, self-testing exercise, attempting to answer questions as though they are part of an actual Board exam. Compare your selected answers against the answers given as "correct" in the Answer Book to assess your level of knowledge and recall of pertinent medical facts and clinical decision-making. Review your results to see your relative strengths and weaknesses by topic areas. Repeat the self-testing process as often as necessary to improve your knowledge and proficiency and ultimately to ensure your mastery of the material.

Author/Editor:
J. Thomas Cross, Jr., MD, MPH, FACP
Vice President, Education
MedStudy Corporation
Colorado Springs, CO

Reviewers:
Robert A. Hannaman, MD
President/CEO
MedStudy Corporation
Colorado Springs, CO

Candace Mitchell, MD
Associate Director, Education
MedStudy Corporation
Colorado Springs, CO

MedStudy Disclosure Policy

It is the policy of MedStudy to ensure balance, independence, objectivity, and scientific rigor in all of its educational activities. In keeping with all policies of MedStudy and the Accreditation Council for Continuing Medical Education (ACCME), any contributor to a MedStudy CME activity is required to disclose all relevant relationships with any entity producing, marketing, re-selling, or distributing health care goods or services consumed by, or used on, patients. Failure to do so precludes acceptance by MedStudy of any material by that individual. All contributors are also required to submit a signed Good Practices Agreement affirming that their contribution is based upon currently available, scientifically rigorous data; that it is free from commercial bias; and that any clinical practice and patient care recommendations offered are based on the best available evidence for these specialties and subspecialties. All content is carefully reviewed by MedStudy's CME Physicians Oversight Council, as well as on-staff proofreaders, and any perceived issues or conflicts are resolved prior to publication of an enduring product or the start of a live activity.

MedStudy Disclosure

MedStudy Corporation, including all of its employees, **does not** have a financial interest, arrangement or affiliation with any commercial entity producing, marketing, re-selling, or distributing health care goods or services consumed by, or used on, patients. Furthermore, MedStudy complies with the AMA Council on Ethical and Judicial Affairs (CEJA) opinions that address the ethical obligations that underpin physician participation in CME: 8.061, "Gifts to physicians from industry," and 9.011, "Ethical issues in CME."

For Further Study

MedStudy Internal Medicine Review Core Curriculum, 14th Edition. MedStudy Corporation, Colorado Springs, CO, 2011.
MedStudy 2011 Video Board Review of Internal Medicine. MedStudy Corporation, Colorado Springs, CO. 2010.
Harrison's Principles of Internal Medicine, 17th Edition. Anthony S. Fauci, Eugene Braunwald, Dennis L. Kasper, Stephen L. Hauser, Dan L. Longo, J. Larry Jameson, and Joseph Loscalzo (eds). McGraw-Hill Medical, 2008.
Cecil Medicine, 23rd Edition. Lee Goldman, MD, and Dennis Arthur Ausiello, MD. Saunders Elsevier, 2008.

Web-based:
National Guideline Clearinghouse:
http://www.guideline.gov/
http://www.ahrq.gov/
American College of Physicians Guidelines: www.acponline.org/clinical_information/guidelines

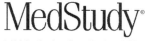

Initial Certification · Recertification · CME

P.O. Box 38148
Colorado Springs, CO 80937-8148
Phone: 1-800-841-0547, ext. 3
FAX: 1-719-520-5973

CME CREDIT APPLICATION

IMPORTANT: You must complete this form and submit it (and the evaluation) to MedStudy to receive CME credit. CME credit is available <u>only</u> to the original purchaser of this product. Issuance of a CME Certificate is subject to verification of product ownership.

CME Credit Application
2011 Internal Medicine Board-Style Questions & Answers
Release Date: December 1, 2010   Expiration Date: December 1, 2013

MedStudy is accredited by the Accreditation Council for Continuing Medical Education (ACCME) to provide continuing medical education for physicians.

MedStudy designates this educational activity for a maximum of 75 *AMA PRA Category 1 Credits*™. Physicians should claim credit only commensurate with the extent of their participation in the activity.

My signature on this document certifies my participation in the MedStudy CME activity: 2011 Internal Medicine Board-Style Questions & Answers (one hour = one credit).

I am claiming _____ *AMA PRA Category 1 Credits*™ (maximum credits: 75).

Signature: _____   **Date**: _____

Printed Name: _____

Street Address: _____

City/State/Zip Code: _____

Telephone: _____   Fax: _____

Permanent E-mail*: _____

Exact name of **original purchaser** (individual or institution)
☐ Same as above ☐ Other_____

Please select the method of delivery for your completed CME certificate. (*E-mail preferred.)

❏ Mail   ❏ Fax   ❏ **E-mail** (Please ensure your e-mail will accept <u>attachments</u> from MedStudy.)

CME processing fee: $40

Payment method: ❏ Check or money order (payable to MedStudy)
                          ❏ Visa ❏MasterCard

FAX to: (719) 520-5973 or Mail to: MedStudy
                                                      P.O. Box 38148
                                                      Colorado Springs, CO 80937-8148

Card # _____Expiration Date _____

Authorized Signature on Credit Card Account _____

The following 2-page evaluation must also be completed and submitted to receive CME credit.

IMPORTANT: EVERY question on this Evaluation MUST be answered.

Specialty: ☐ IM   ☐ IM/Peds   ☐ Other: _____

How did you hear about this product?
☐ Catalog   ☐ Colleague   ☐ MedStudy Website   ☐ Internet Search   ☐ Medical Meeting   ☐ Other

Which of the following BEST describes your use of this product?
☐ Prepare for Initial **Certification**   ☐ Prepare for **Recertification** (MoC)   ☐ **General Review/Reference**

How many years have you been out of residency?
☐ Still a Resident   ☐ < 1 yr   ☐ 1–7 yrs   ☐ 8–14 yrs   ☐ 15–20 yrs   ☐ > 20 yrs

When did you most recently take (or will you take) your ABIM exam?
Year_____ Spring___ Summer___ Fall ___

Did you pass the ABIM exam?
☐ Yes   ☐ No   ☐ Don't know yet   ☐ Haven't taken it yet   ☐ Didn't use product for exam prep

Please rate the following regarding your use of this product:

	STRONGLY DISAGREE				STRONGLY AGREE
The content presented met my personal educational expectations	1	2	3	4	5

Due to my learning with this product, I am able to …

Integrate and demonstrate increased overall knowledge of Internal Medicine	1	2	3	4	5
Identify and remedy areas of weaknesses (gaps) in knowledge and clinical competencies	1	2	3	4	5
Describe the clinical manifestations and treatments of diseases encountered in Internal Medicine and effectively narrow the differential diagnosis list by utilizing the most appropriate medical studies	1	2	3	4	5
Apply the competence and confidence gained through participation in this activity to both a successful Board exam-taking experience and daily practice	1	2	3	4	5
Question and Answer exercise format was a viable mode of instructional delivery	1	2	3	4	5
The content was free of pharmaceutical bias	1	2	3	4	5
The content offered a reasonable balance of diagnostic and therapeutic options	1	2	3	4	5

Please rate the quality of coverage for the following specialty/subspecialty areas:

	POOR		FAIR		EXCELLENT
Allergy & Immunology	1	2	3	4	5
Cardiology	1	2	3	4	5
Dermatology	1	2	3	4	5
Endocrinology	1	2	3	4	5
Gastroenterology	1	2	3	4	5
Hematology	1	2	3	4	5
Infectious Disease	1	2	3	4	5
Miscellaneous	1	2	3	4	5
Nephrology	1	2	3	4	5
Neurology	1	2	3	4	5
Obstetrics/Gynecology	1	2	3	4	5
Oncology	1	2	3	4	5
Ophthalmology	1	2	3	4	5
Pulmonary Medicine	1	2	3	4	5
Psychiatry	1	2	3	4	5
Rheumatology	1	2	3	4	5

Did this product help you identify and remedy any gaps in medical knowledge and/or clinical judgment skills?

❑ Yes
❑ No

If yes, please elaborate:

After you used this product, were you able to apply any of what you learned to daily practice?

❑ Yes
❑ No

If yes, please elaborate and be as specific as possible?

Were there specific topic areas that you feel were not adequately covered in this product?

❑ Yes
❑ No

If yes, please elaborate and be as specific as possible:

General comments about this product, your Board exam experience, or suggestions for improvement

Thank you for completing this Evaluation.

MedStudy®

Internal Medicine Board-Style Questions & Answers

2011

Questions

Edited by J. Thomas Cross, Jr., MD, MPH, FACP

TABLE OF CONTENTS

Note: Many of the images you see throughout this Questions book can be viewed in color in the image atlas at the back of the book.

Disclaimers

IMPORTANT: These Q&A books are meant to be used as an adjunct to the MedStudy Internal Medicine Review Core Curriculum. The ABIM exams cover a vast realm of diagnostic and treatment knowledge. Board-simulation exercise such as these self-testing Q&As are valuable tools, but these alone are not adequate preparation for a Board exam. Be sure you use a comprehensive IM review resource in addition to these Q&As for adequate exam preparation.

Content. The primary purpose of this activity is educational. Medicine and accepted standards of care are constantly changing. We at MedStudy do our best to review and include in this activity accurate discussions of the standards of care, methods of diagnosis, and selection of treatments. However, the authors/presenters, editors, advisors, and publisher—and all other parties involved with the preparation of this work—disclaim any guarantee that the information contained in this activity and its associated materials is in every respect accurate or complete. MedStudy further disclaims any and all liability for damages and claims that may result from the use of information or viewpoints presented. We recommend you confirm the information contained in this activity and in any other educational material with current sources of medical knowledge whenever considering actual clinical presentations or treating patients.

ABIM. For over 20 years, MedStudy has excelled in determining and teaching what a clinically competent Internal Medicine physician should know. The American Board of Internal Medicine (ABIM) tests this exact same pool of knowledge. MedStudy's expertise, demonstrated by the superb pass rate of those who use it in their studies, is in the actual "teaching" of this knowledge in a clear, learner-friendly manner that results in a stronger knowledge base, improved clinical skills, and better Board results. Although what we teach is in sync with what the Boards test, MedStudy has no affiliation with the ABIM, and our authors, editors and reviewers have no access to ABIM exam content. Our material is developed as original work by MedStudy physician authors, with additional input from expert contributors, based on their extensive backgrounds in professional medical education. This content is designed to include subject matter typically tested in certification and recertification exams as outlined in the ABIM's publicly available exam blueprints but makes no use of, and divulges no details of, ABIM's proprietary exam content.

A note on editorial style: MedStudy follows a standardized approach to the naming of diseases, using the non-possessive form when the proper name of a disease is followed by a common noun. So you will see phrasing such as "This patient would warrant workup for Crohn disease" (as opposed to "Crohn's disease"). Possessive form will be used, however, when an entity is referred to solely by its proper name without a following common noun. An example of this would be "The symptoms are classic for Crohn's." Styles used in today's literature can be highly arbitrary, some using possessive and some not, but we believe consistency is important. It has become nearly obsolete to use the possessive form in terminology such as Lou Gehrig's disease, Klinefelter's syndrome, and others. *The AMA Manual of Style, JAMA,* and *Scientific Style and Format* are among the publications that are now promoting and using the non-possessive form. We concur with this preference.

MEDSTUDY
P.O. Box 38148
Colorado Springs, CO 80937-8148
(800) 841-0547

About the questions and answers in this learning activity

The questions, answers, and explanations in this learning activity are developed by the author, based on his own background of 20 years in professional medical education and his ongoing consultation with many subspecialty experts from around the country. Dr. Cross is also an author/editor for MedStudy's Internal Medicine Board Review Core Curriculum and a teacher at MedStudy's live Internal Medicine Certification and Recertification Board review courses. He has previously been an associate professor in the Departments of Internal Medicine and Pediatrics at Louisiana State University Health Sciences Center and is a past president of the National Internal Medicine/Pediatrics Program Directors' Association. Dr. Cross is Board Certified in Internal Medicine, Pediatrics, and in both Adult and Pediatric Infectious Disease (ID).

Knowing the importance that the IM Boards place on established standards of care, having researched recent and pertinent practice guidelines, and having reviewed the publicly available ABIM Board exam blueprints, Dr. Cross is well aware of the areas of knowledge most likely to be tested on today's Board exams. As a result, you will find that the percentage of questions by topic in this activity mirrors the Board template. You will find questions of varying length here. The very short ones are designed to nail home an important point you need to know and remember for your Boards. The lengthier questions help you integrate content on a subject with additional clinical information to better simulate a real-life patient scenario.

This helps you recognize disease states and associated treatment, which is a skill heavily tested on Board exams. Some selected patient case scenarios may appear more than once, or with only slight variations, with the associated questions addressing different diagnosis and treatment aspects of the case. This is in keeping with the approach Board questions take in limiting patient case assessments to one key testing point.

In short, this Q&A material is designed to impart not only relevant knowledge for IM Board exams but also challenge your skills in interpretation and intervention, which is what Board exams attempt to assess. Which is why we call these, appropriately, "Board-style" questions and answers.

There is a popular misconception that members of organizations perceived to be associated with medical boards write Board exam questions. E.g., ACP/MKSAP with the American Board of Internal Medicine or AAP/PREP with the American Board of Pediatrics. Not only is this not true, it is actually forbidden for anyone to write formal Board exam questions if they work for a company or organization in the business of producing Board preparation materials. This would compromise the integrity of the examining process.

MedStudy is proud to be able to bring you Board-style questions and answers of the highest quality—to offer you education that is relevant in a format that reinforces your knowledge to prepare you well for whatever challenge the ABIM Board exam presents you. One final note: Even the best question and answer exercise by itself is not an adequate preparation for a Board exam. These Q&As should be used as an adjunct to a comprehensive Board review course (such as MedStudy's Internal Medicine Board Review Core Curriculum). The Boards cover a vast realm of information that Board simulation Q&As alone cannot encompass.

GASTROENTEROLOGY

1.

A 23-year-old man comes to your office with complaints of intermittent dysphagia. He says it occurs after swallowing a large amount of food—especially if he takes a big bite of steak and doesn't chew it very well. It has never occurred with liquids. The dysphagia occurs every 1–2 months and then goes away. He has had some heartburn in the past but none recently. He denies chest pain, nausea, vomiting, or sore throat.

Social History: He works as an auto mechanic and is a non-smoker.

Family History: Family history is significant for no known malignancies.

Which of the following tests listed would be the most appropriate diagnostic test?

   A. Upper endoscopy.
   B. *H. pylori* testing.
   C. Manometry.
   D. 24-hour pH probe.
   E. No procedure is indicated.

2.

A 68-year-old woman presents with complaint of difficulty swallowing. She notes that about 4 months ago she had trouble swallowing big pieces of food; this has progressed to the point that she has difficulty swallowing thick liquids now. She has lost about 10 pounds and attributes this to a lack of desire to eat. She denies heartburn or other symptoms.

Past Medical History: Significant for 2 packs of cigarettes per day for 40 years.

Physical Exam: She is alert and oriented to person, place, and time. She is pale in appearance. She has indeed lost 12 pounds since you last saw her. Otherwise, her examination is normal.

Which of the following is the most probable etiology of her weight loss and dysphagia?

   A. Schatzki ring
   B. Squamous cell carcinoma of the esophagus
   C. Adenocarcinoma of the esophagus
   D. Achalasia
   E. Peptic stricture

3.

A 42-year-old man presents with difficulty swallowing solid food. He says that the symptoms began over 3 years ago. In the beginning, he noted it only with trying to swallow large pieces of steak without chewing properly. Since then, it has gradually worsened to the point that he must chew each piece of food carefully and use lots of water to swallow. He has not had weight loss. He denies fever or night sweats. He has not had any nausea, vomiting, or recent abdominal pain.

Social History: He does not smoke and does not drink alcohol.

Which of the following is the likely etiology of his dysphagia?

    A. Achalasia
    B. Schatzki ring
    C. Peptic stricture
    D. Adenocarcinoma of the esophagus
    E. Squamous cell carcinoma of the esophagus

4.

A 28-year-old female has a long history of alternating diarrhea and constipation. This has been present since college, although there are times when symptoms are worse than other times. It has not been progressive in any way. She also has diffuse lower abdominal cramps that are associated with the loose stools. She admits that symptoms can be worse with stress. She had a colonoscopy 1 year ago, which was normal.

Past Medical History: Negative.

Social History: The patient has a stressful job that keeps her very busy. She frequently eats fast food because of her busy schedule.

Family History: Positive for Crohn disease in 1 cousin

Review of Systems: She denies any weight loss. She has never had overt bleeding. The diarrhea never wakes her at night.

Physical Examination: Completely unremarkable. The abdomen is soft and nontender without any organomegaly. The patient does bring records with her from her prior medical care.

Which of the following is the most appropriate next step?

    A. Repeat colonoscopy, because something like inflammatory bowel disease might have been missed.
    B. Reassure patient and start with a high-fiber diet along with referral to a stress management clinic.
    C. 72-hour fecal fat test.
    D. Referral to psychiatry.

5.

A 30-year-old male presents for a routine examination. He has no specific complaints. He has just moved to the area with his job.

Past Medical History: Negative, and his only medications are multivitamins. He exercises daily and doesn't smoke cigarettes or drink alcohol.

Family History: He notes that his father had colon cancer at age 55, and in fact, he is now undergoing chemotherapy. He had a paternal uncle who died from colon cancer at age 42. His brother, who is 35 years old, recently had a colonoscopy, at which time several polyps were removed. The patient doesn't know the histology of those polyps, just that they were small.

Which of the following studies would you recommend?

A. Colonoscopy now
B. Flexible sigmoidoscopy now combined with fecal occult blood testing every year and a colonoscopy at age 40
C. Colonoscopy at age 40
D. Air-contrast barium enema now

6.

A 25-year-old woman has a 3-year history of diarrhea and abdominal cramping. These symptoms seem to worsen with stress, but the diarrhea can wake her. She was told she had irritable bowel syndrome and was placed on a high-fiber diet. She was also given dicyclomine as an antispasmodic agent. However, her symptoms did not improve with these methods, and she is seeking another opinion.

Past Medical History: Negative, and her only medicine is dicyclomine.

Family History: Negative.

Social History: Unremarkable.

Review of Systems: Significant for a 4-lb. weight loss in the past 3 months. She denies any fever or chills.

Physical Examination: She is in no apparent distress.
HEENT: Unremarkable.
Chest: Clear.
Cardiac: Normal.
Abdomen: Nondistended with normal bowel sounds. She does have focal tenderness with some degree of fullness in the R lower quadrant.

You order a colonoscopy, and the colon is normal until entering the right colon. At this point, one sees numerous shallow ulcers. The ileum is edematous with multiple shallow ulcers. Biopsies of these areas reveal chronic inflammation and ulceration. Some of the biopsies from normal tissue adjacent to the ulcers come back with normal histology without any significant inflammation.

The most appropriate treatment at this time would be which of the following?

A. Infliximab 300 mg infused over 2 hours
B. Azathioprine 50 mg PO once daily
C. Mesalamine 400 mg PO tid
D. Prednisone 40 mg qd with a taper of 10 mg every week

7.

A 60-year-old woman presents with a sudden onset of cramping abdominal pain. This pain is in the lower abdomen and was associated with passing several maroon stools. The pain is severe, but intermittent. All of these symptoms started 4 hours ago. She has never had symptoms like these before.

Past Medical History: Significant for CAD. She has had several stents placed. She is on daily aspirin. She quit smoking 20 years ago and does not drink alcohol.

Review of Systems: She has always had normal bowel movements in the past. She denies any syncope, chest pain, or recent weight loss.

Physical Examination: She is in mild distress, but mostly resting comfortably.
Her HR is 100 and BP is 120/60.
Skin: Normal
HEENT: Unremarkable and sclera are anicteric. There is no lymphadenopathy.
Cardiac Exam: Normal
Chest: Clear
Abdomen: She demonstrates mild tenderness in the LLQ. There is no hepatomegaly. The abdomen is not distended, and bowel sounds are normal. There is no mass present.
Rectal Exam: Maroon stool is present.

Laboratory: Hgb 11.6, WBC 7,200, PT 12, INR 1

What is the next appropriate test?

  A. Mesenteric angiography
  B. Flexible sigmoidoscopy
  C. CT scan of abdomen and pelvis
  D. Upper GI small bowel series

8.

A 29-year-old female with long-standing Crohn disease presents to the Urgent Care Clinic after being awakened from a sound sleep with the sudden onset of RUQ pain. She has never had a pain like this and says this is clearly different from what she has experienced with her Crohn disease in the past. The pain lasted 1 hour. It is now gone. It was constant for the entire hour. She vomited twice and obtained relief after the second episode. She had Crohn disease diagnosed 10 years ago. She had a resection of the R colon and terminal ileum 7 years ago. Approximately 5 years ago, it was documented that she had recurrent disease to the ileum. An upper GI demonstrated extensive ileal involvement at that time. She was placed on mesalamine. Since that time, she has done well with only rare episodes of mild abdominal pain. Her baseline is 3 stools per day, and this has not recently changed.

Past Medical History: Significant only for the Crohn disease. Only medication is mesalamine 400 mg, which she takes 6 times a day.

Social History: Unremarkable.

Family History: She has a maternal aunt who has Crohn disease.

Physical Examination: She is in no apparent distress although somewhat tired from the lack of sleep. She is afebrile. Vital signs are normal.
HEENT: Unremarkable
Chest: Clear
Cardiac Exam: Normal
Abdomen: Nondistended. There is slight tenderness in the RUQ without hepatomegaly. There are no palpable masses.
Rectal Exam: Done, but there was no stool present.

Laboratory: Bili 1.0, AST 42, ALT 36, amylase 85, WBC 9,200, Hgb 12.

You recommend which of the following?

A. Gallbladder ultrasound
B. EGD
C. Upper GI small bowel series
D. Intravenous Pyelogram (IVP)

9.

A 35-year-old male has a new-onset diarrhea, which started 3 days ago. Initially it was watery stool but then, 2 days ago, he started passing blood as well. He has had associated abdominal cramps and nausea. He has vomited once as well. He was previously normal and has never had any significant gastrointestinal symptoms in the past.

Past Medical History: Unremarkable

Social History: He denies any foreign travel. He has no history of recent antibiotics. He has a hectic schedule and frequently eats fast-food hamburgers, almost on a daily basis.

Family History: Negative for inflammatory bowel disease or any other significant GI disease.

Review of Systems: Does admit to feeling weak. He denies any fever or chills.

Physical Examination:
HR 100, BP 100/60.
Skin turgor is slightly decreased and mucous membranes appear dry.
There is no lymphadenopathy.
Pulmonary and cardiac exam: Normal
Abdomen: Nondistended. Bowel sounds are hyperactive. No rushes or tinkles. He is slightly tender in the RLQ although without a palpable mass.

Laboratory: Hgb 16, WBC 12,000.

A number of stool studies have been drawn. Routine cultures, including *Salmonella* and *Shigella*, are negative. He is positive for *E. coli* O157:H7. Currently there are pending tests of the stool for *Clostridium difficile* toxin and ova, cysts, and parasites.

Which of the following antibiotics would you recommend?

A. Ciprofloxacin 500 mg bid x 7 days
B. Amoxicillin-clavulanic acid (Augmentin®) 875 mg bid x 10 days
C. Metronidazole 500 mg tid x 10 days
D. No antibiotic treatment

10.

A 40-year-old woman has suffered with chronic heartburn and diarrhea for 2 years. She takes over-the-counter omeprazole, which gives some relief of the heartburn. She also complains of chronic diarrhea, with 5 to 6 loose bowel movements a day and some epigastric discomfort. EGD is done and shows grade III esophagitis. Multiple shallow ulcers are seen in the duodenal bulb and second portion of the duodenum.

You recommend which of the following?

A. Continue omeprazole, but add sucralfate qid.
B. Continue omeprazole, but add metoclopramide before meals.
C. Order *H pylori* ELISA.
D. Order fasting serum gastrin after stopping the omeprazole for 7 days.

11.

A 68-year-old Caucasian female presents to her primary care physician with a chief complaint of weakness and fatigue. This has been present for 2 months, although she initially attributed this to the stress of the holidays. She has always been healthy and active. She denies any abdominal pain, change in bowel habits, chest pain, or pulmonary symptoms. However, she does admit to some dyspnea on exertion.

Past Medical History: Otherwise healthy. Her only medication is estrogen replacement. She has had a remote hysterectomy.

Family History: Unremarkable

Social History: Unremarkable

Review of Systems: She denies any melena or rectal bleeding. She has occasional nocturnal reflux after a late meal, but this happens only once a month and has been completely relieved by OTC famotidine.

Physical Examination: She is somewhat pale, but in no apparent distress.
HEENT: Unremarkable. There is no lymphadenopathy.
Chest: Clear
Cardiac Exam: Normal
Abdomen: Soft and nontender. There are no palpable masses. There is no enlargement of liver or spleen.
Rectal Exam: Stool is brown and heme-positive.

Laboratory: Hgb 9.6, MCV 72, LFTs are normal.

Which of the following should you order next?

A. EGD
B. Tagged RBC bleeding scan
C. Colonoscopy
D. Upper GI small bowel series

12.

A 36-year-old male presents to your office. He is new to the area and wants to establish himself with a new physician. He feels fine and has no specific complaints. His past medical history is remarkable, and he comes in wondering if he does need some sort of evaluation. As a teenager, he was diagnosed as having familial polyposis coli. Both his father and his older brother have the disease as well. At age 20, he underwent a total abdominal colectomy with an ileorectostomy, and he has done well ever since. He has 4 bowel movements a day, and this has been a constant feature since the surgery. There has been no change in his pattern of bowel movements. He denies any overt rectal bleeding.

Past Medical History: Otherwise healthy.

Family History: As mentioned.

Social History: Negative for cigarettes and alcohol.

Review of Systems: Denies abdominal pain or symptomatic reflux.

Physical Examination: Remarkably healthy male with a well-healed midline abdominal incision.

Laboratory: All normal including Hgb of 14.2.

You schedule the patient for a flexible sigmoidoscopy, which reveals 10 polyps in the residual rectum. All of the polyps are less than 1.0 cm. All are removed by snare technique, and the subsequent pathology reveals them to be adenomatous polyps. There is no significant dysplasia or carcinoma found in any of the specimens.

At this time, you recommend which of the following studies?

    A. X-rays of the mandible to rule out osteoma.
    B. Upper endoscopy.
    C. CT scan.
    D. No further studies. Simply repeat the flexible sigmoidoscopy in 1 year.

13.

A 24-year-old woman complains of malaise for the past 2–3 months. She is on no medications, and her past medical history is otherwise normal.

Family History: Significant for mother who has Hashimoto disease.

Social History: Works as a legal secretary and does not drink alcohol or smoke cigarettes.

Review of Systems: She denies any fever, chills, jaundice, abdominal pain, or itching.

Physical Examination: The patient is comfortable.
HEENT: Unremarkable. No lymphadenopathy.
Skin: Anicteric. No signs of spider angiomas.
Chest: Clear to auscultation.
Cardiovascular Exam: Normal
Abdomen: Liver is slightly enlarged, 3 cm below the right costal margin, and slightly tender. The abdominal exam is otherwise normal. There is no enlargement of the spleen.

Laboratory: AST 1,020, ALT 1,220, bili 1.0, alk phos 120.

You order subsequent liver tests that come back as follows:
Anti-smooth muscle antibody positive 1:250
Antimitochondrial antibody positive 1:40
HCV Ab positive
HCV RNA negative
HBsAg negative
HBcAb negative
HAV Ab negative

You order a liver biopsy, which does show chronic active hepatitis.

Which of the following would be the next best treatment?

    A. Start treatment with oral prednisone and azathioprine 50 mg a day.
    B. Start treatment with ursodeoxycholic acid 250 mg bid.
    C. Start treatment with interferon and ribavirin.
    D. Start treatment with pegylated alpha-interferon.

14.

A 60-year-old woman presents with acute-onset RUQ pain and fever. She has had prior episodes of self-limited pain that never lasted more than 30 minutes. She has now been in pain for 2 hours. PMH is negative. No medications. ROS: slight darkening of urine.

Physical Examination: T 100° F, HR 100, BP 130/80; tender RUQ without peritoneal signs

Laboratory: HGB 15, WBC 16,000, T Bili 3.0, AST 120, ALT 110, Alk Phos 400
Amylase and lipase NL

Ultrasound: Gallbladder has many stones. No gallbladder wall thickening.
Dilated common bile duct with several apparent stones.

You start her on antibiotics.

Based on what you know, which of the following would be the next best course of action?

    A. ERCP
    B. MRCP
    C. EGD
    D. Abdominal CT scan

15.

A 17-year-old female presents for evaluation of chronic abdominal pain. She describes the pain as a chronic, colicky pain in the right lower quadrant. She has had no weight gain for a year and has delayed puberty.

Physical Examination: Thin, pale adolescent. She has no secondary sexual development. Her abdomen is slightly distended. There are good bowel sounds but mild tenderness in the right lower quadrant and a palpable loop of bowel. The stool from the rectal tests is heme-positive.

The stool has red and white blood cells. The stool cultures, O&P, and *C. difficile* toxin are all negative.

Which of the following studies is most likely to confirm your diagnosis?

    A. Upper gastrointestinal series with small bowel follow-through
    B. Barium enema
    C. Upper and lower endoscopy with mucosa biopsy
    D. Abdominal CT scan

16.

A 16-year-old male presents with the "flu" and jaundice. The parents seem unconcerned by the jaundice. They relate that he "does this" every time he becomes ill. In fact, his father and uncle do the same thing. You convince them to check their son's bilirubin, which comes back with indirect bilirubin of 4 mg/dL. The remainder of the liver tests are normal, as is a complete blood count.

Which of the following would be the next appropriate step?

    A. Liver biopsy
    B. Reassurance that this is a benign condition
    C. Liver ultrasound
    D. Hepatitis panel

17.

A 60-year-old Caucasian male presents to your office with a chief complaint of dysphagia. Dysphagia has been present for about 2 years. He notes difficulty swallowing both solids and liquids, which has been slightly progressive over the 2-year period. He also notes some nocturnal regurgitation. His primary care doctor saw him a year ago and gave him omeprazole. However, this has not improved the symptoms.

Past Medical History: Remarkable for coronary artery disease and cardiomyopathy, with an ejection fraction of 20%. He's had a CVA in the past although no residual impairment. He also has a long history of COPD due to both past and current cigarette use.

Upper GI is ordered, which demonstrates a dilated esophagus that is tapered at the junction to the stomach. EGD shows the same findings. There is a dilated esophagus with retained food and smooth tapering at the distal esophagus. There is no evidence of any mass effect at the distal esophagus. The stomach and duodenum are normal.

Which of the following is the best treatment recommendation for this individual?

    A. Botox injection into the lower esophageal sphincter
    B. Laparoscopic myotomy
    C. Pneumatic dilatation
    D. Bougie dilatation
    E. Esophageal resection

18.

A 40-year-old female patient routinely sees a rheumatologist for scleroderma. She now complains of new-onset dysphagia. Actually, the symptoms have been gradually increasing over the past 4 to 6 months. She denies any prior heartburn or nocturnal regurgitation. The dysphagia is present for meats and breads. It has never been noted for liquids.

Past Medical History: Significant only for the scleroderma.

Review of Systems: Significant for no weight loss or chest pain.

Physical Examination: Remarkable for the typical findings of scleroderma on the face and hands.

You recommend which of the following?

A. Avoid endoscopy because of increased risk of perforation in scleroderma.
B. Empiric use of omeprazole and re-evaluate in 2 months.
C. Empiric metoclopramide before meals because of the likelihood that gastroparesis is a factor in reflux.
D. EGD and dilate if there is a narrowed area of the esophagus.

19.

A 28-year-old Internal Medicine resident has been healthy all of his life. He recently developed acne, which was attributed to the copious ingestion of Hershey bars on call nights. He prescribed for himself doxycycline. He presents now with a sudden onset of pain with swallowing anything, either liquid or solid. This has been present for 2 days. He is weak and is having difficulty sleeping because of the discomfort. He has rarely suffered heartburn in the past. His physical exam is significant for the moderate distress and some blood-shot eyes from lack of sleep.

You recommend which of the following?

A. EGD
B. Trial of proton pump inhibitor
C. Hyoscyamine PO before meals
D. Upper GI, x-ray, and HIV assay
E. Supportive care

20.

A 60-year-old Caucasian male has a long history of reflux symptoms. Most of these symptoms are well controlled with omeprazole every morning. He also has adult-onset asthma, and this is, in fact, the biggest problem for this patient at this time. The asthma started at about the age of 40. It has progressively worsened and is difficult to control with inhalant therapy. He has required frequent courses of prednisone, but he is becoming less responsive to this therapy as well.

Social History: The patient has a good diet without any bad habits.

Review of Systems: Positive for nocturnal regurgitation and occasional waking with choking sensation.

Upper GI series shows a small hiatal hernia and reflux.
EGD: Demonstrated linear esophageal erosion but no suspicion of Barrett esophagus.

Which of the following treatments do you recommend?

A. Empiric fluconazole for possible candida esophagitis.
B. Increase the omeprazole to twice a day.
C. Evaluate for anti-reflux surgery.
D. Intensify the asthma regimen with chronic steroids.
E. Add an H_2 blocker at bedtime to the morning proton pump inhibitor.

21.

A 55-year-old male complains of upper abdominal discomfort and fullness after meals. He also has frequent belching. These symptoms have been present for several months. He gives no prior history of similar symptoms. The symptoms have been persistent despite the use of his wife's prescription of famotidine 20 mg twice a day for the last 8 weeks.

Past Medical History: Significant for hypertension. His only medication is benazepril. He denies any aspirin or NSAID use.

Review of Systems: Negative for weight loss

Physical Examination: Reveals a benign abdomen.

Upper GI has been performed and shows a gastric ulcer of benign appearance.

Which of the following is the most appropriate next step?

    A. Empiric omeprazole and re-evaluate in 8 weeks
    B. EGD now
    C. Continue famotidine for 8 more weeks
    D. CT scan

22.

A 35-year-old Caucasian female has had Crohn disease since age 19. She has had one prior surgery, which was the resection of the cecum and terminal ileum at age 23. She has required a number of tapering courses of prednisone in early years but only twice in the past 5 years. She describes 2–3 soft stools per day. She has occasional abdominal cramps. She considers herself fairly well controlled right now with regard to the Crohn disease. Her current medication is mesalamine 2.4 g/day.

Review of Systems: She denies any joint or bone pain. She does not have fever. Her weight is stable.

Physical Examination: There is slight fullness in the right lower quadrant without a definite mass.

Colonoscopy last year demonstrated recurrent disease at the anastomosis, extending about 15 cm into the ileum.

Which of the following would be the most appropriate next step at this time?

    A. Bone mineral density now.
    B. Bone mineral density at age 40, but for now maximize calcium intake.
    C. Empiric weekly alendronate.
    D. Initiate azathioprine and, 3 months later, check bone mineral density.

23.

A 40-year-old male has had ulcerative colitis since age 25. He has been having one or two flares per year. He moved to your city 5 years ago and has not established himself with a doctor. He has been using the prednisone prescription from his last physician for his rare flares. He was told at his last colonoscopy 5 years ago that his colitis involved the entire colon. He currently has normal bowel movements and denies any blood or mucus.

Past Medical History: Is otherwise healthy.

Social History: He smokes a cigar nightly and works as a stockbroker.

Review of Systems: Negative for joint pain or mouth ulcers.

Physical Examination: Completely normal.

Which of the following do you recommend?

    A. Colectomy because of the cancer risk after 15 years of pancolitis.
    B. Quit smoking because it will help his colitis.
    C. Start sulfasalazine 2 g/day.
    D. Start azathioprine for steroid-sparing effects.

24.

A 70-year-old woman presents with a 6-month history of watery diarrhea. Previously, she always had normal bowel movements. She describes mild cramping and abdominal pain. Neither the pain nor the diarrhea wakes her up at night. She denies weight loss.

Past Medical History: Significant for hypothyroidism. Her current medications include thyroid replacement and ibuprofen.

Review of Systems: Positive for chronic joint pain relative to degenerative joint disease.

Social History: She has had no recent antibiotics. Her only travel history is a once-a-year trip to Branson, Missouri, to hear Wayne Newton sing.

Initial workup revealed normal CBC, TSH, and comprehensive metabolic panel. The stool was negative for WBC, negative for blood, negative for fat stain, negative for *Giardia* antigen. The measured stool output was 500 g/day.

Which of the following tests should you order next?

    A. Upper GI small bowel series
    B. Endoscopy with small bowel biopsy
    C. Colonoscopy with biopsy
    D. CT scan of the abdomen

25.

A 32-year-old male patient is new to town and seeks your advice as his new physician. He was diagnosed as having familial polyposis coli at age 16 and had a total colectomy with ileorectostomy at age 19. He has done well since that time. He has 3 bowel movements a day.

Family History: Remarkable in that his father and two brothers have polyposis and have all had colectomies. His grandmother died of colon cancer at the age of 40.

He has a flexible sigmoidoscopy and many small adenomatous polyps are completely removed. A recent EGD for occasional reflux symptoms was performed. There were multiple large polyps in the body and fundus of the stomach. The duodenum had several tiny, white plaques. One of these plaque-like lesions was biopsied, revealing an adenoma. No dysplasia was found.

Because a duodenal adenoma was found, you recommend which of the following?

   A. Video capsule to look at the rest of the small bowel.
   B. Nothing for now but repeat EGD in 1–2 years.
   C. Repeat EGD to remove as many of the gastric polyps as possible with a snare technique.
   D. Surgery to remove the stomach and duodenum.

26.

A 25-year-old college student (7th year senior) presents to a local Emergency Department due to passing a large, bloody, maroon stool. He has no abdominal pain but does feel lightheaded. This is his third admission in 2 years for a similar episode. His last episode was 6 months ago, at which time he required 4 units of transfused RBCs because his hemoglobin dropped to 6 gm. At that time, he had a normal colonoscopy for both the colon and the terminal ileum. There were no diverticula present on exam. Upper endoscopy was also performed and was normal. Prior to that bleed, he had frequent headaches caused by studying so much. For the past 6 months, he has not taken any NSAIDs. Since that last bleed, he has also had a normal upper GI small bowel series. A [99m]technetium pertechnetate scan is done and confirms your diagnosis.

Past Medical History: Otherwise normal

Physical Examination: His heart rate is 120 and BP 90/60. His abdominal exam is normal. His stool is maroon and bloody. His initial hemoglobin is 8.8 gm.

Of the following, which should you do next for this patient?

   A. Angiography.
   B. CT abdomen.
   C. Surgery.
   D. Prep with Go Lightly® and repeat colonoscopy.

27.

A 65-year-old woman presents to the office with the complaint of fatigue for 2 months. She has no specific pain or discomfort. She has noted no change in her bowel habits.

Past Medical History: Significant for hypertension and hyperlipidemia. She avoids aspirin and NSAIDs.

Family History: Non-contributory.

Physical Exam: This is unremarkable except for the presence of heme-positive brown stool.

Laboratory: Hemoglobin is 7.8 with an MCV of 65.

You refer to the local gastroenterologist, who does an EGD. The EGD is normal. A colonoscopy is also performed. Unfortunately, she had a very tortuous colon, and the exam was only to the hepatic flexure. The patient was then sent back to you for consideration of additional studies.

Given what you know now, what should you do next for this patient?

    A. Send for colonoscopy to a different gastroenterologist.
    B. Upper GI small bowel series.
    C. No further studies; start the patient on iron and have her return to clinic in 2 months for a repeat hemoglobin check.
    D. Air contrast barium enema.

28.

A 27-year-old woman presents with a 3-month history of rectal bleeding, abdominal cramps, and diarrhea. Colonoscopy was performed, leading to a diagnosis of ulcerative colitis. She is started on mesalamine at a dose of 2.4 g/day. There is some initial improvement in her symptoms, but 3 weeks later, she develops a different abdominal pain: a severe epigastric pain that radiates to the back. The pain is associated with nausea and vomiting. She came to the Emergency Department, where her amylase was found to be 3,000 with a lipase of 2,400. Acute pancreatitis was diagnosed. The patient was made NPO, an NG tube was placed, and IV fluids were administered. Mesalamine was stopped. The ultrasound done at that time showed a normal gallbladder. After 5 days in the hospital, the patient was discharged with resolution of her symptoms and a normal amylase and lipase. Two weeks later the patient again presents to the Emergency Department with epigastric pain. This is somewhat similar to her past pancreatitis but not as severe. Amylase is 300 and lipase is 280. CT scan shows a 4-cm cyst in the body of the pancreas.

Which of the following do you recommend?

    A. ERCP now to rule out common bile duct stone
    B. Interventional radiology to drain the pseudocyst
    C. Surgery now to remove the cyst and the gallbladder
    D. Treat with conservative measures like bowel rest and IV fluids

29.

A 68-year-old male has been in the ICU for 2 weeks with a very complicated story. He was originally admitted to the hospital for elective resection of a colon cancer of the cecum. Within the first three days after surgery, this was complicated by an aspiration pneumonia and acute respiratory failure, requiring intubation and mechanical ventilation. He also developed acute renal failure and a prolonged ileus, requiring the patient to be on TPN for nutrition.

During this time, the patient has been kept on broad-spectrum antibiotics, including ticarcillin/clavulanic acid and gentamicin. The abdomen has been distended the entire period. The patient is unable to complain since the day they started ventilatory support. Now after one week of being afebrile, the patient has a fever to 102° F. Abdominal ultrasound shows a gallbladder with a thickened wall and a small amount of fluid around the gallbladder. No stones are seen.

Laboratory: Bilirubin is 1.6, AST 110, and ALT 90.

Given this scenario, which of the following is the most appropriate next step?

A. Interventional radiology to place a percutaneous cholecystostomy drainage tube.
B. ERCP and stent placement.
C. Laparoscopic cholecystectomy.
D. Change antibiotics to cover potential fungal sepsis.

30.

A 60-year-old former rock and roll guitarist presents to your office for a checkup. He tried to donate blood and was told he may have hepatitis. He has no specific complaints and denies jaundice or pruritus.

Past Medical History: Significant for depression; treated with paroxetine.

Review of Systems: Negative

Social History: He admits to some past intravenous drug use but none in the last 20 years. He drinks beer only on Sundays because he watches Detroit Lions football games.

Physical Exam: There are multiple tattoos seen; he has no enlargement of liver or spleen. There is no ascites, and he is anicteric.

Laboratory: AST 20, ALT 18
Bilirubin 0.2, alkaline phosphatase 65
HCV antibody positive, HB surface antigen negative, HB core antibody negative.

The AST and ALT are checked again 2 weeks later and remain within normal limits.

You recommend treatment with which of the following?

A. Pegylated interferon.
B. Ribavirin.
C. No treatment at this time.
D. You bring out your old set of drums from the attic and start practicing and offer to form a new group with your patient.

31.

A 24-year-old male presents to the ED with symptoms of esophageal food impaction for 2 hours after eating chicken. He is salivating and spitting up frothy secretions. He can't drink water without regurgitating. This is his 4th episode of these symptoms. He denies heartburn. PE is normal. Labs and CXR are okay.

What is next appropriate step?

A. GI consult for EGD to remove food bolus
B. Barium swallow
C. CT of chest
D. Surgery consult

32.

A 70-year-old Asian male who hasn't seen a doctor in 20 years comes to your office. No significant history; he is brought in by family who reports that the patient is not eating and is losing weight. Patient says he has progressive difficulty swallowing. Six months ago, he could swallow soft foods, but now it is slow even getting liquids down. There is a long history of cigarettes and alcohol.

Exam shows muscle wasting. Labs are significant for Hgb of 10 and MCV 72. A barium swallow shows a 3 cm segment of severe narrowing of the distal esophagus.

Which is the next best step in the management of this patient?

A. Give samples of a PPI
B. Esophageal motility study
C. Refer to GI for EGD
D. Calcium-channel antagonist

33.

A 70-year-old patient presents with hematemesis and melena. There is no prior history of gastrointestinal bleeding, and these symptoms started one hour before arrival in the Emergency Department. There is no prior history of abdominal symptoms or heartburn.

Past Medical History: Significant for mild hypertension and hyperlipidemia.

Social History: Unremarkable

Family History: Non-contributory

Review of Systems: There is a long history of osteoarthritis, for which the patient takes ibuprofen on a regular basis. There's been no recent weight loss. He was weak and lightheaded on admission, but this is now improved.

Physical Examination: On arrival to the Emergency Department, BP was 100/60, HR 120. Now, after IV fluids, the BP is 130/80 and HR 96. The patient is comfortable and not in apparent distress. Cardiac and pulmonary exams are otherwise normal. The abdomen is soft and nontender. A nasogastric tube is in place and coffee ground-like material is aspirated.

Laboratory: Hgb 10 and hematocrit 30. INR is normal. The other labs are unremarkable.

Upper endoscopy reveals a 2-cm ulcer in the antral region of the stomach. There is a raised protuberance within the ulcer crater. Initially, a blood clot was attached to it, but the blood clot was easily removed by lavage. There is a large volume of blood in the fundus of the stomach. There are several other non-bleeding erosions in the antrum as well as the duodenum.

Which is the next best step in the management of this patient?

    A. Endoscopic treatment with a heater probe applied to the visible vessel.
    B. Refer to surgery.
    C. Interventional angiography with selective cannulization and embolization of the celiac artery.
    D. High dose of intravenous proton pump inhibitor.
    E. Keep the nasogastric tube in and use titrated antacid to maintain a neutral pH.

34.

A 60-year-old patient has been suffering with diarrhea for the past 2 years. She has undergone extensive evaluation, which has been negative. She's had 2 colonoscopies, including one with random biopsies, both of which were negative and otherwise unrevealing. The diarrhea is described as up to 6 watery bowel movements per day. It has been somewhat progressive over the past 2 years. 3 days ago, the patient started having nausea and profuse vomiting to the point that she could not hold down any food.

Past Medical History: Otherwise unremarkable. The patient is not on any medications.

Review of Systems: Positive for a long history of heartburn, for which the patient takes antacids and over-the-counter H_2 blockers. There has been 10-lb weight loss in this past year.

Social History: Negative

Family History: Negative

Physical Exam: This is pertinent for the patient being in mild-to-moderate distress. Hemodynamically, the patient is now stable after being in the hospital for the past 2 days with IV fluids. Abdominal exam is normal.

Because of the nausea and vomiting, the patient underwent an upper endoscopy. This revealed severe ulcer esophagitis. There was a large volume of secretions within the stomach. The pH of this fluid was 1.0. There were multiple ulcers present in the duodenum, including the descending portion of the duodenum.

Laboratory: Tests on arrival include Hgb 10 and hematocrit 30; transaminases were normal. Electrolytes were normal. Fasting serum gastrin was 5,000. ELISA *H. pylori* antibody was negative. An abdominal CT scan was negative for any tumor or mass within the abdominal cavity or liver.

Based on these findings, which of the following would you recommend next?

    A. Exploratory laparotomy.
    B. Endoscopic ultrasound.
    C. Vagotomy and antrectomy.
    D. Chemotherapy to include 5-fluorouracil.
    E. Start infusion with octreotide.

35.

A 30-year-old woman has long-standing Crohn disease. She had one prior surgery 3 years ago, at which time 24 inches of the ileum and cecum were removed. She has had no other surgeries and takes mesalamine 1.6 gm each day. There has been no evaluation in the past 3 years. She comes into the office with 2 months of intermittent RLQ pain and loose stools. She denies fever, nausea, or vomiting. Exam reveals tenderness in RLQ but without mass. CBC and LFTs are normal.

Which of the following is the most likely diagnosis for this patient?

A. Primary sclerosing cholangitis
B. Gallstones
C. Kidney stones
D. An exacerbation of Crohn disease

36.

A 35-year-old woman presents with a chief complaint of belching and indigestion. When she says "indigestion," she means that there is some substernal discomfort that can actually be present all day long. She doesn't have pyrosis or regurgitation. It's never a burning type pain. She's had these symptoms for 2 years but says they are getting worse and unbearable. She is constantly belching; even during the interview she belches several times a minute. She also complains of some abdominal distention but no severe abdominal pain. Bowel movements are, for the most part, normal.

Past Medical History: Unremarkable except for hysterectomy and a cholecystectomy performed for a poorly functioning gallbladder. Current medications include esomeprazole 40 mg PO bid. She has been on this for one month and can't say that it helps the symptoms even to a small degree.

Social History: The patient does not smoke cigarettes or drink alcohol. She is married and works as a real estate agent. Family history is negative for any gastrointestinal disease. Review of systems is otherwise negative.

Physical Exam: The patient does not appear in acute distress although she is belching frequently. There are no other abnormalities on exam.

Past workup includes upper endoscopy, which demonstrated normal esophagus without any gross reflux esophagitis. She had a 24-hour ambulatory esophageal pH recording, which demonstrated that she had 20 episodes of acid reflux over 24 hours. All of these were brief in duration, lasting less than a minute. Her total time with a pH less than 4 was less than 1%.

Based on these findings, which of the following should you do next?

A. Evaluate for an acid hypersecretory condition like Zollinger-Ellison syndrome.
B. Double the current dose of proton pump inhibitor to esomeprazole 80 mg bid.
C. Consider a psychiatric referral or the use of anti-anxiety medicine.
D. Add metoclopramide 4 times a day.
E. Consider surgery for an anti-reflux procedure.

37.

A 27-year-old woman has had Crohn disease for the past 5 years. She is hospitalized now for the 3rd episode of small bowel obstruction in the past 6 months. In between episodes she feels well, although she has to avoid any foods containing fiber or else she will experience abdominal cramps and distention. She has not had diarrhea, and she's maintained her weight. The prior two episodes of obstruction have been treated with hospitalization, IV fluids, IV steroids, and NG suction. Each hospitalization was about 5 days and resolved such that she was discharged on a tapering dose of prednisone.

Past Medical History: Significant for the Crohn disease, as mentioned. She's had no other complications from the Crohn disease. She is on azathioprine 100 mg a day for the past 2 years. She cannot tolerate infliximab or similar agents. She is also on mesalamine 2.4 gm per day. She's been on prednisone in various doses, 4 out of the last 6 months.

Review of Systems: Pertinent for occasional joint pain. She denies any mouth lesions or painful eye conditions. Family history is negative for inflammatory bowel disease.

Social History: Positive for cigarette use, smoking 1 pack a day.

Colonoscopy done one year ago revealed the colon to be free of any active Crohn disease. The terminal ileum was stenotic and would not allow passage of the scope into the ileum. The patient had an upper GI small bowel series after her second episode of obstruction, revealing a tight 10-cm area in the distal ileum.

Based on these findings, which of the following would be the best plan of action?

- A. Increase her dose of azathioprine to 150 mg/day.
- B. Schedule the patient for colonoscopy and balloon dilation of the stricture.
- C. Increase the mesalamine dose to 4 g/day.
- D. Add metronidazole 500 mg PO tid.
- E. Refer for surgical resection of the terminal ileum.

38.

A 25-year-old woman whom you've been following for the past 4 years for ulcerative colitis comes to the office with the joyful news that she and her husband are expecting their first child. She's 8 weeks pregnant at this time. She has had ulcerative colitis since the age of 20. A past colonoscopy demonstrated this is distal disease, or proctosigmoiditis. She has had approximately 2 or 3 flares of disease activity each year, each time being manifest as frequent bloody stools with mucus and tenesmus. During those times she has responded to oral prednisone added to her regimen of mesalamine. Previously she was on 1.6 g/day of mesalamine. Over the past 6 months this was increased to 3.2 gm of mesalamine/day, and this is seen to benefit her with fewer flares of the colitis.

Past Medical History: Otherwise unremarkable

Review of Systems: Negative for joint pain, skin lesions, mouth lesions or painful eye lesions

Physical Exam: Normal

For this patient with ulcerative colitis and new pregnancy, which of the following would be the most appropriate treatment?

 A. Continue mesalamine in its current dose.
 B. Discontinue the mesalamine and initiate low dose prednisone 10 mg/day.
 C. Add azathioprine to the mesalamine with the hopes of preventing any flares during pregnancy.
 D. Continue mesalamine in the same dose and add 20 mg prednisone/day.
 E. Schedule colonoscopy to determine the disease activity prior to any changes in therapy.

39.

A 16-year-old male presents to the Emergency Department with a 3-day history of diarrhea. The diarrhea was initially watery but has now become bloody. Over the past day he's had vomiting as well. He reports diffuse abdominal cramps and discomfort. He's never had any condition like this in the past.

Past Medical History: Otherwise negative

Social History: Unremarkable

Family History: Unremarkable

Review of Systems: He denies any joint pain or fever.

Physical Exam: He appears to be in moderate distress with a resting heart rate of 100. His skin turgor is decreased, and his mucous membranes seem dry. His abdomen is slightly distended, and there seems to be some mild tenderness in the right side of the abdomen.

Laboratory: Hgb 13, WBC 14,500. Stool is negative for *Campylobacter, Salmonella*, and *Shigella* but positive for *E. coli* O157:H7.

The patient is at risk for which of the following complications?

 A. Guillain-Barré syndrome
 B. Hemolytic uremic syndrome
 C. Encephalopathy
 D. Peripheral neuropathy
 E. Aplastic anemia

40.

A 40-year-old woman presents to your office with complaint of acute diarrhea. She works as an attorney, providing mostly pro bono work for an inner city legal aid office. The diarrhea has been present for about a year but has been getting worse over the past couple of months such that it has interfered with her appearances in court. She describes 5–6 watery, occasionally foul-smelling stools per day. She never wakes with bowel movements. This is not associated with any abdominal cramps, only some urgency.

Past Medical History: Otherwise unremarkable

Social History: Of interest—she spent two years in Indonesia working in rural communities as a teacher. She also lived in Mexico City for about 6 months. She had a brief stay in Rwanda in her campaign to save the mountain gorillas. She does not smoke cigarettes or drink alcohol. She does not take any medication.

Physical Exam: The skin exam is normal. There is slight thickening and redness of her tongue. There is no lymphadenopathy. Heart, chest, and lung exam is normal. Abdomen is slightly distended with increased gurgling and mild tympany. There is no hepatomegaly or palpable masses. Extremities are normal.

Laboratory: Tests reveal Hgb 13, MCV 108. WBC and platelets are normal. The albumin is normal at 4.0, but a calcium level is slightly depressed at 7.5. B_{12} level is normal, and folate level is significantly depressed. Initial stool for ova and parasites is negative.

Based on these findings, which of the following is the most appropriate therapy?

- A. Trial of tetracycline
- B. Trial of metronidazole
- C. A gluten-free diet
- D. Trial of pancreatic enzymes
- E. Lomotil (diphenoxylate)

41.

A 55-year-old woman presents to the Emergency Department with the onset of moderately severe abdominal cramping associated with the passage of a maroon, bloody stool. This occurred suddenly earlier in the day without any prior symptoms. Since then she's had two additional passages of maroon stool, each time associated with significant cramps.

Past Medical History: Significant for stable coronary artery disease. She has two stents in place but has good function and is active and free of angina. She takes a daily aspirin.

Review of Systems: Otherwise negative

Social History: She is active without any smoking or alcohol history.

Family History: Negative for any significant gastrointestinal disease

Physical Exam: The patient is in moderate distress, clutching her abdomen. She is afebrile with normal vital signs. The abdomen is slightly tender to palpation in the left lower quadrant with increased bowel sounds overall.

The patient is started on IV fluids. Sigmoidoscopy is performed, which reveals a normal rectum. However, 25 cm from the anus in the sigmoid colon, there is an abrupt transition into colonic mucosa that is so edematous that a lumen cannot be identified. The mucosa is purple with what looks like submucosal hemorrhage. These changes are circumferential but begin very suddenly with an immediate transition to a normal mucosa distally.

Based on this endoscopic appearance and clinical presentation, the best treatment at this time would be which of the following?

- A. Intravenous hydrocortisone
- B. Intravenous metronidazole
- C. Oral mesalamine
- D. Surgical resection, subtotal colectomy
- E. Medicated cortisone enemas

42.

A 78-year-old nursing home patient presents with a readmission to the hospital for diarrhea. She was hospitalized one month ago and was found to have stool that was positive for *C. difficile* toxin. She was treated with metronidazole but experienced severe nausea and vomiting. She was sent home on this regimen, but, according to the nursing home staff, she was unable to complete her course of therapy because of the vomiting. The frequency of the stools improved but never returned to baseline. The diarrhea became worse the day prior to admission.

Past Medical History: Significant for several cerebrovascular accidents in the past. She has recurrent urinary tract infections that have required numerous courses of antibiotics over the past 2 years. She has limited activity. She is able to feed herself without assistance. She enjoys watching "Wheel of Fortune" each evening.

Physical Exam: She is in no apparent distress. The exam is unremarkable for this elderly woman. Abdomen is slightly distended but without tympany. The bowel sounds seem hyperactive. Initial studies show stool that is positive for fecal leucocytes as well as positive for the toxin for *C. difficile*. Her WBC count is 16,500.

Based on these findings, which of the following regimens would be most appropriate next course of action?

- A. Vancomycin 250 mg PO qid x 14 days
- B. A regimen of probiotics
- C. Intravenous metronidazole in conjunction with promethazine (Phenergan®) to prevent the vomiting
- D. Amoxicillin with intravenous gentamicin
- E. Intravenous fluid with oral mesalamine

43.

A 50-year-old male presents to the Emergency Department after 3 large, maroon stools have been passed. The patient has no prior history of gastrointestinal bleeding. There have been no associated cramps, abdominal pain, or discomfort. The patient admits to being slightly lightheaded but mostly scared.

Past Medical History: Negative except for mild hypertension. The patient takes an aspirin a day for general cardiac protection, although he's never been told that he's at risk for cardiac disease.

Family History: Negative for any gastrointestinal problems

Social History: Unremarkable

Review of Systems: Significant for the lack of any other positive symptoms

Physical Exam: The patient is resting comfortably. HR 90, BP 130/90. Skin is normal. Abdomen is soft and nontender. Bowel sounds are normal. There is no enlargement of the liver or spleen. No palpable masses.

Based on the history, which of the following is the most likely cause of this patient's bleeding?

- A. Diverticulosis
- B. Arteriovenous malformations (AVMs)
- C. Ischemic colitis
- D. Ulcerative colitis
- E. Infectious colitis

44.

A 24-year-old male, currently in his 6ᵗʰ year in college, describes intermittent diarrhea for 3 years. The loose stools can alternate with constipation. He never has nocturnal stools. He suffers with mild abdominal cramps. PMH is negative.

Review of Systems: Negative for weight loss, fever, joint pain, skin rash

Social History: Beer on weekends, 2 glasses milk each day. He constantly chews diet gum. No travel.

Which of the following is the best plan of action at this time?

    A. 72-hour fecal fat collection
    B. Colonoscopy
    C. CT of abdomen and pelvis
    D. Trial of lactose-free, sorbitol-free diet

45.

A 35-year-old woman and mother of 3 children presents with a chief complaint of constipation. The constipation has been present for a number of years. She remembers taking laxatives while in college. The constipation has become more of a problem over the past couple of years. She has taken a variety of over-the-counter laxatives, which do provide her some relief. She has about 2 bowel movements per week and describes the stool as hard to pass. She never has alternating diarrhea or severe abdominal pain, but she does have some abdominal distention.

Past Medical History: Unremarkable except for three uncomplicated pregnancies. Her diet is irregular because she has been trying to lose weight. She often skips breakfast and has a Slim-Fast for lunch. Her evening meal is often spent eating leftovers from the children's meals.

Social History: Negative for alcohol or tobacco intake

Family History: Negative for any significant gastrointestinal disease

Physical Exam: Unremarkable

Laboratory: CBC and TSH are both within normal range. A barium enema reveals possibly a few diverticula within the sigmoid colon but is otherwise normal.

Based on these findings, which of the following interventions do you recommend?

    A. A regimen of fiber supplementation and increased water intake
    B. Tegaserod 6 mg PO bid
    C. Metoclopramide 10 mg PO qid
    D. Fleets enemas every third day
    E. Lactulose 30 cc PO bid

46.

A 60-year-old gentleman presents to the Emergency Department with his 3rd episode of melena. The first episode was 3 years ago and the patient had, according to history, a negative workup at an outside hospital. The 2nd episode, six months ago, did not prompt him to go to the hospital, and it resolved spontaneously. He thought that it was wise to get this third episode checked out. He describes a two-day history of dark, tarry stools. He denies any hematemesis or abdominal pain. At no time has he had maroon stools. This is similar to the past episode. He does feel a little bit weak but not lightheaded.

Past Medical History: Otherwise negative

Family History: Both his father and his paternal uncle were plagued by recurrent gastrointestinal bleeding. He is not aware of a diagnosis made in either one of them. The father ended up dying from lung cancer.

Review of Systems: Significant for recurrent epistaxis in his 20s

Physical Exam: Reveals a male in no apparent distress. Skin exam is normal except for some faint telangiectasias on the lips and fingertips. On examination of the nasal mucosa, there appear to be some telangiectasias as well. The mouth exam is otherwise normal; there is no lymphadenopathy. No spider angiomas are seen on the chest. Chest and lung exam are otherwise normal. The abdomen is soft and nontender. The stool is heme-positive with melena.

On admission to the hospital, the initial Hgb is 11. INR is normal. Endoscopy reveals 4 well-defined erythematous lesions within the stomach that are felt to be arteriovenous malformations (AVMs). Another 3 similar lesions were seen in the duodenum. The patient also had colonoscopy, which showed sigmoid diverticulosis but no other vascular malformations.

Based on these findings, which of the following is the most likely diagnosis?

A. Peutz-Jeghers syndrome
B. Familial polyposis
C. Osler-Weber-Rendu syndrome
D. Diverticular bleeding
E. Celiac sprue

47.

A 24-year-old male presents to the Emergency Department with a 2-day history of severe nausea, vomiting, diarrhea, and fever (temperature up to 101° F). Before this illness, he was healthy and active without any underlying medical problems. His girlfriend, who is a nurse, brought him to the ED when she suspected that he was dehydrated. He does not take any medications on a regular basis, although for the past few days he has been taking up to 8 extra strength acetaminophen (500 mg) per day.

Family History: Unremarkable

Social History: Significant for unprotected sex with several females over the past 4 years. He does describe ingestion of raw oysters one week prior to admission. He consumes alcohol—3 beers per week.

Physical Exam: The patient is in moderate stress. BP 100/70, HR 100. His skin turgor is decreased. There is obvious scleral icterus on exam. Cardiac and lung exam is otherwise normal. The abdomen is soft and non-distended with normal bowel sounds. Extremities are normal.

Laboratory: Significant for WBC 5,500 and Hgb of 15.5. The differential is normal. Total bilirubin is 4. AST 30, ALT 28, alkaline phosphatase 90, INR 1.

Which of the following is the most likely explanation for the patient's jaundice?

    A. Gilbert syndrome
    B. Hepatitis A
    C. Hepatitis B
    D. Acetaminophen toxicity
    E. Autoimmune chronic active hepatitis

48.

The father of a family calls the Emergency Department at midnight with a query for advice and gives the following scenario. The entire family, within a one-hour time period, noted the onset of profuse vomiting. Each person had multiple episodes of retching. The persons involved include the husband, wife, and two teenage children. The husband and wife have started to manifest some diarrhea as well. No one has a fever, although each person does have some abdominal cramps. None has any underlying medical illnesses, nor have they experienced anything like this before.

On further review, we find that both teenagers had eaten fast-food hamburgers and french fries for lunch. The entire family went to a Chinese food restaurant that evening. The wife mentions that she threw out some mayonnaise from the refrigerator that smelled bad the day before.

Which of the following is the most likely cause of the described illness?

    A. Food poisoning with *Staphylococcus aureus*
    B. Food poisoning with *B. cereus*
    C. *Salmonella*
    D. *E. coli* O157:H7
    E. Viral gastroenteritis

49.

A 54-year-old former rock and roll musician presents to your office because "I need my liver checked out." 10 years ago, he was told that he had hepatitis C. He received interferon treatment for the first 6 months but has not had follow-up since that time. He says that he feels fine except for occasional weakness. He denies ever having jaundice or confusion. He denies abnormal swelling or weight loss.

Past Medical History: Otherwise negative

Social History: The first line of the question says it all! He denies any ongoing alcohol intake or use of illicit drugs.

Review of Systems: He denies any chest pain, shortness of breath, melena, change in bowel habits or abdominal pain. He has gained 10 lbs in the past year.

Physical Exam: The patient is well nourished. There is no jaundice. There are no spider angiomas on physical examination. Lungs are clear and cardiac exam is normal. The liver is 2 cm below the right costal margin, and the spleen tip is palpable. There may be trace ascites present and there is no edema found.

Laboratory: Tests reveal Hgb 12, WBC 7,200, platelet count 98,000. Bilirubin 2, AST 56, ALT 50, alkaline phosphatase 100, INR 1.1. An upper endoscopy is recommended, and this reveals large, grade IV esophageal varices. Some of the varices have red markings over them. There is no active bleeding. There are no definite varices in the stomach, although the stomach has an erythematous mosaic pattern.

Based on the endoscopic findings, which of the following should you do next?

    A. Initiate propranolol and titrate the dose until the patient has a heart rate of < 60.
    B. Endoscopic sclerotherapy with repeat exam until the varices are obliterated.
    C. Initiate spironolactone therapy 50 mg PO bid.
    D. No therapy for now, but repeat endoscopy in 6 months to assess varices.
    E. Start lactulose 30 cc bid.

50.

A 55-year-old male is in for an executive health check. He has no specific complaints and is not taking any medications. He doesn't have any family history of colon cancer. As part of the exam, you recommend a screening colonoscopy and this was performed. On this exam, a 1.2-cm polyp in the ascending colon was removed with snare technique. The pathology of the polyp showed a tubular adenoma with low-grade dysplasia. The patient now asks you when he should have a follow-up colonoscopy.

Which of the following recommendations do you give the patient regarding follow-up colonoscopy?

    A. 1 year.
    B. 3 years.
    C. 5 years.
    D. 10 years.
    E. No follow-up is needed.

51.

Brendan Kelly is a 22-year-old man with a negative past medical history. He presents with the chief complaint of "turning yellow." He noticed that he was becoming yellow in the eyes yesterday. Today, he noted that his skin was also yellow. He has no nausea, vomiting, or other complaints.

Past Medical History: Negative

Social History: Works at Taco Ringer as a cook. Lives with his girlfriend of 3 months. Became sexually active and had multiple sexual partners starting one year ago. Has been monogamous for 3 months and 1 day. Regular on the Larry Stinger Show. Smokes marijuana on weekends. Drinks two or three 6-packs of beer on weeknights.

Family History: Mother, 36, is pregnant. Father, 38, is in prison for selling fake Madonna concert tickets. Sister, 12, with attention deficit disorder.

Review of Systems: Essentially noncontributory

Physical Exam: Only pertinent findings: Scleral icterus; liver edge down about 3–4 cm with a span of 12 cm, slightly tender; spleen tip palpable; no spider angiomas

Laboratory:
Anti HAV IgM Positive
Anti-HBc IgM Negative
Anti-HBc IgG Negative
HBsAg Negative

How do you interpret the laboratory data?

A. He has acute hepatitis A and past infection with hepatitis B.
B. He has acute hepatitis A.
C. He has chronic hepatitis A and acute hepatitis B.
D. He has acute hepatitis A and chronic hepatitis B.
E. He has neither hepatitis A nor hepatitis B.

52.

All of the following are indications for colonoscopy except:

A. Bright red blood on toilet paper in an 18-year-old college student
B. Gross lower gastrointestinal bleeding in a 30-year-old man
C. *Streptococcus bovis* bacteremia in a 60-year-old woman
D. Hemoccult positive screen in a 60-year-old woman
E. Iron deficiency anemia in a 45-year-old man

53.

For the following table, which choice indicates hepatitis B infection that has resolved?

Table of hepatitis B serology:

Option	HBsAg	HBcAb (IgG)	HBsAb
A	Negative	Positive	Positive
B	Negative	Negative	Positive
C	Positive	Positive	Negative
D	Negative	Negative	Negative
E	Positive	Positive	Positive

54.

Which of the following causes of diarrhea will typically have fecal leukocytes?

A. *Cryptosporidia*
B. Toxigenic *E. coli*
C. Giardiasis
D. *Shigella*
E. Rotavirus

55.

Four people arrive at the Emergency Department, all within 30 minutes of each other, presenting with similar symptoms. They all describe the sudden onset of nausea and severe vomiting. Shortly thereafter, all of them developed profuse diarrhea and now all complain of severe weakness. All 4 people had been together that afternoon—because they all work for a company in Colorado Springs that provides study materials for doctors taking board exams. The company was celebrating the summer with a picnic. There were a variety of different foods that were brought by different people, including deviled eggs, ham sandwiches, sashimi, barbecue chicken, hamburgers on the grill as well as raspberries and melon balls. None of the people involved remembers eating any other items. All had been swimming in a creek, and 2 admit to possibly ingesting some of the creek water. The nausea started almost exactly 4 hours after the picnic.

On presentation to the Emergency Department, the person complaining of the most profound weakness has a blood pressure of 80/40 with a heart rate of 140 and decreased skin turgor. Temperature is 97° F. Abdomen is soft and nontender. IV fluids have been started.

Which of the following is true?

A. Antibiotic therapy is not indicated.
B. This is probably *Salmonella* related to undercooking of poultry.
C. This is likely giardiasis from drinking the creek water in Colorado.
D. This is likely *E. coli* O157:H7 related to undercooked hamburger.
E. Knowing the strange habits of the people who work for this company, exposure to iguanas is likely and *Salmonella* is a concern.

PULMONARY MEDICINE

56.

Sam B. is a 60-year-old nurse at a local hospital. He has had annual tuberculin skin testing for 10 years. His last PPD a year ago was 5 mm. Today he presents at 72 hours for reading of his PPD placed earlier in the week. He is healthy and denies any health problems; particularly no fevers, sweats, or weight loss.

This is an employee health check, and therefore no physical exam or other information is obtainable.

Laboratory:
PPD at 72 hours: 16 mm
CXR: Normal

Based on the data presented, which of the following should be done next?

  A. Start INH 300 mg daily for 9 months
  B. No treatment because he is older than 35 years old
  C. 4-drug therapy because he is high risk, being in a hospital environment
  D. If he is also HIV positive, you would start INH 300 mg daily for 12 months
  E. Repeat PPD in 2 weeks; if still positive, then start therapy

57.

A 30-year-old female with asthma presents to your office for routine followup. She is currently using her albuterol inhaler 2–3 times/week and is waking from sleep about once/week needing a treatment. She is not on any long-term therapy. She has never been hospitalized and usually does well using albuterol until she gets a cold, at which time she has moderate to severe exacerbations. On physical examination today she is stable with no wheezes. Her peak flow is in the green zone.

How would you change her daily therapy?

  A. Continue current regimen but give oral steroids every time she gets a cold
  B. Add daily inhaled corticosteroids
  C. Add inhaled steroids only during a cold
  D. Do not change anything
  E. Change the albuterol to a long-acting beta-agonist

58.

Cathy H. is a 15-year-old who hunts ducks regularly in northern Louisiana and southern Arkansas. She comes to you with a 2-month history of cough and recent development of hemoptysis. On talking to her, you discover that she has lost 8 pounds in the last month.

Past Medical History: Negative

Social History: Lives in Start, Louisiana, with her mother and father
    Denies use of alcohol

No illicit drug use

Family History: Father died at age 45 of lung cancer
    Grandmother died at age 46 of lung cancer

Physical Examination: BP 100/70, P 95, Temp 100° F, RR 25, Weight 110 lbs.

HEENT: PERRLA, EOMI
TMs: Clear
Throat: Clear

Neck:	Supple
Heart:	RRR without murmurs, rubs, or gallops
Lungs:	Scattered crackles in the bases
Abdomen:	No hepatosplenomegaly
Extremities:	Draining pustular lesion noted on her left arm

She reports that it has been there for 1 month; puts "poultice" on it and it gets better, then it gets worse again.

Laboratory:
    CXR: Possible mass noted at left base
    Gram stain of left arm lesion's fluid: Mixed bacterial flora
    KOH of left arm lesion's fluid: Small budding yeasts
    Acid-fast smear of left arm lesion's fluid: No organisms seen

Based on your findings, which of the following is the most likely diagnosis?

   A. Coccidioidomycosis
   B. Blastomycosis
   C. Histoplasmosis
   D. Tuberculosis
   E. Lung carcinoma

59.

A 65-year-old man is sent to you by his orthopedist, Dr. Butch Bonehead, for pre-op clearance prior to elective hip surgery. The patient has a history of smoking 2 packs a day but quit in his early 30s. He has occasional asthma. He uses a steroid inhaler bid and has to use his albuterol inhaler only once a week.

His physical examination is significant for a left-sided limp. His respiratory rate is 15/minute. He has a few scattered end-expiratory wheezes on chest examination. The remainder of his examination is normal.
A peak-flow is done in the office and is 91% of his predicted value.

What is/are the most appropriate step(s) to take prior to clearing him for surgery?

   A. Pulmonary consultation.
   B. Spirometry before surgery.
   C. Spirometry and arterial blood gases with a carboxyhemoglobin level.
   D. He is of high operative risk and you refuse to clear him for surgery.
   E. No further pulmonary testing is needed; he may go to surgery.

60.

A 25-year-old pregnant woman (at 22 weeks) presents for evaluation with dyspnea and pleuritic type chest pain. She says that she has had progressive leg swelling for the past 6 days. A room air ABG is obtained and shows: pH 7.48, $PaCO_2$ 23, PaO_2 80.

What is the best diagnostic test to do at this point?

A. V/Q scan
B. Bilateral venography
C. Duplex ultrasonography
D. Pulmonary angiography
E. D-dimer

61.

A 60-year-old man presents to your office for routine yearly follow-up. He has mild hypertension for which he takes lisinopril. He is otherwise healthy. He denies cough or shortness of breath. He used to smoke 1 ppd of cigarettes for 20 years but quit 6 years ago. He works in a manufacturing plant, and as part of the yearly physical, he underwent Pulmonary Function Tests. The results are as follows: FEV_1/FVC 65%, FEV_1 2.4 L (82% predicted). There was no bronchodilator response. A chest radiograph was read as "unremarkable."

Which one of the following recommendations would be most appropriate for this patient?

A. Start long-acting beta-agonist twice daily
B. Initiate pulmonary rehab program
C. Vaccinate for influenza annually
D. Start nocturnal oxygen
E. Start long-acting anti-cholinergic agent once daily

62.

A 52-year-old female was evaluated for a lung mass three months ago. This was biopsied via bronchoscopy, and pathology was consistent with lung adenocarcinoma. After further evaluation, she was determined to have Stage IIIB lung carcinoma. She has completed her first cycle of combined chemotherapy and radiation therapy. Today, she complains of a one-week history of right lower extremity edema and pain, as well as a sudden onset left-sided pleuritic chest pain associated with shortness of breath. Her vitals are as follows: HR 120 bpm, RR 24, oxygen saturations 92% RA, blood pressure 125/80. Duplex ultrasonography of the right leg reveals an occlusive thrombus of the right common femoral vein. Serum creatinine level is 2.1.

Which of the following is the next appropriate action?

A. Obtain V/Q scan
B. Start LMWH at treatment dosing alone
C. Start LMWH at treatment dosing with concomitant warfarin
D. Obtain chest CT angiogram
E. Start infusion of thrombolytic agent

63.

A 45-year-old female presents to the Emergency Department with a seven-day history of progressive shortness of breath. She was seen earlier this week by her primary care provider, who ordered a chest radiograph. This revealed a hazy area of infiltration in her right lower lobe, and he started a quinolone antibiotic. Upon presentation to the ED four days later, she was noted to be in severe respiratory distress with a respiratory rate of 45, HR of 130, and oxygen saturations of 78% on 4 L oxygen. She was promptly intubated and placed on mechanical ventilation. Chest radiograph revealed bilateral alveolar infiltrates throughout the entire lung fields. Her BNP level was normal, and an echocardiogram revealed normal LV function and moderately elevated pulmonary artery pressures. Currently she is on FiO_2 of 100%. Her ABG reveals a PaO_2 of 90 mmHg. Blood cultures grew *Streptococcus pneumoniae*. She has now been admitted to the intensive care unit.

Which of the following interventions has been shown to reduce mortality in patients with this disease process?

A. Use of prone positioning
B. Initiation of mechanical ventilation with tidal volumes set at 4–6 mL/kg of ideal body weight
C. Initiation of mechanical ventilation with tidal volumes set at 8–10 mL/kg of actual body weight
D. Use of continuous narcotic infusion to improve ventilator synchrony
E. Use of pulmonary artery catheter to measure pressures to guide further management

64.

A 40-year-old woman with sarcoidosis that is under fairly good control comes in today for a routine checkup and is noted to have a BP of 150/95. In reviewing her file, you note that the last time she came in she also had an elevated BP, and you had recommended dietary changes as well as weight loss. She has attempted these but evidently will require a pharmacologic agent to control her hypertension. Her current routine laboratory studies are normal.

Which of the following is the best agent for her to use?

A. Thiazide diuretic
B. Loop diuretic
C. Fosinopril
D. Atenolol
E. Calcium channel blocker

65.

A 42-year-old female complains of exertional dyspnea for about 2 years that seems to be gradually progressing. She now has difficulty doing simple household chores without dyspnea. She has no associated cough, sputum, fever, chills, or wheezing. She has occasional episodes of feeling lightheaded with exercise but no palpitations. She has no significant past medical history and takes no medications except for a multivitamin. She is a lifelong non-smoker. Physical exam reveals normal vitals except a resting oxygen saturation of 89%. Lungs are without abnormal sounds. Cardiovascular exam reveals a 2/6 holosystolic murmur at the left mid-sternal border, an RV impulse at the left sternal border, and A_2 and P_2 sounds that are equal in intensity. Pulmonary function tests only reveal a reduced DLCO, which is 45% predicted. Chest radiograph is normal. Echocardiogram reveals normal left ventricular function but is notable for right atrial and ventricular dilatation, 3+ tricuspid regurgitation, and an estimated pulmonary artery systolic pressure of 84 mmHg. Right heart catheterization is performed, which estimated the mean pulmonary artery pressure to be elevated at 55 mmHg. Pulmonary capillary wedge pressure is normal. Chest angiogram is without pulmonary embolus. Serologic testing for connective tissue disease is all negative.

Which one of the following is <u>not</u> currently used for treatment in patients with this clinical entity?

A. Warfarin
B. Oral endothelin receptor antagonist
C. Oral cyclophosphamide daily
D. Oxygen therapy
E. Subcutaneous prostacyclin therapy

66.

A 55-year-old woman presents to your office for evaluation of dyspnea. She has no cough or chest pain and complains of shortness of breath with exertion only. No nocturnal symptoms. She has occasional episodes of near syncope but no palpitations. Chest radiograph doesn't reveal any abnormalities. Pulmonary Function Tests are ordered.

	Actual	Predicted %
FVC (L)	4.88	122
FEV_1 (L)	3.09	126
FEV_1/FVC	.63	82
TLC (L)	6.17	107
RV (L)	1.41	81
DLCO	12	50

Based on her DLCO result, which of the following is unlikely?

A. Emphysema
B. Pulmonary arterial hypertension
C. Anemia
D. Erythrocytosis
E. Pulmonary embolus

67.

A 60-year-old man with COPD on chronic bronchodilator therapy and theophylline visits a local "doc-in-the-box" and receives a prescription for an antibiotic for "bronchitis." He begins his medication but 3 days later returns to you with nausea, vomiting, and tremulousness.

Which of the following is the likely explanation for his new symptoms?

A. The antibiotic he was given was amoxicillin.
B. The antibiotic he was given was cefazolin.
C. The antibiotic he was given was gatifloxacin.
D. The antibiotic he was given was ciprofloxacin.
E. He stopped taking his theophylline.

68.

You are visiting your cousin who is a news reporter in New York City for the *National Expose*, a "tell-all" entertainment rag that has been threatened by terrorist groups in recent weeks. Your cousin is concerned about bioterrorism agents and asks if he should be worried about a "severe pneumonia" diagnosed in one of his colleagues.

Which of the following organisms can be spread from person to person in respiratory droplets from a person with pneumonia and is useful as a bioterrorist agent because of this characteristic?

    A. *Yersinia pestis*
    B. *Bacillus anthracis*
    C. *Clostridium botulinum*
    D. *Neisseria morphagenesis*
    E. *Arcanobacterium haemolyticum*

69.

You are presented a patient with respiratory problems. Her PFT patterns are as follows:

Reduced expiratory flows
Increased total lung capacity
Reduced vital capacity
Mild increase in DLCO
Significant response to bronchodilator

Based on the above results, which of the following diagnoses is most likely?

    A. COPD
    B. Emphysema
    C. Interstitial lung disease
    D. Asthma
    E. Sarcoidosis

70.

On the Board examination, a series of pleural effusions are presented to you.

Which of the following is most consistent with an effusion due to rheumatoid arthritis?

    A. Pleural fluid white cell count of 15,000
    B. Pleural fluid glucose > 80 mg/dL
    C. Pleural fluid glucose < 30 mg/dL
    D. Pleural fluid pH < 7.0
    E. Pleural fluid triglyceride > 115 mg/dL

71.

A 70-year-old man with COPD has had worsening shortness of breath for the last 6 months. He cannot move from his chair to his refrigerator without stopping several times along the way to catch his breath. A resting ABG is obtained and reveals the following:

pH: 7.46
PCO_2: 50
PaO_2: 50
HCO_3: 32
O_2 sat: 84%

Based on his history and laboratory results, what do you recommend?

A. He should be placed on oxygen therapy when he has exertion.
B. He should be placed on oxygen therapy during the daytime.
C. He should be placed on oxygen therapy 24 hours/day.
D. He should not be placed on oxygen therapy except for episodes of shortness of breath.
E. He cannot be placed on oxygen therapy because his ventilatory drive will be impaired.

72.

A 60-year-old woman with lung cancer presents with new onset of anisocoria. Her right pupil is much smaller and rounder than her left pupil. You dim the lights in the examination room and note that the left pupil has dilated much more.

On examination, her right pupil responds briskly to light. She has mild ptosis on the right and anhidrosis on the right as well. Her right pupil constricts with pilocarpine administration, and dilates with atropine. However, when you apply 4% cocaine, it minimally dilates.

Where is her likely abnormality located?

A. Left optic nerve
B. Right optic nerve
C. Left sympathetic chain
D. Right sympathetic chain
E. Left occipital lobe

73.

A 32-year-old man presents with pleural effusion and cough. He was released from prison 4 months ago and has been living on the streets of Miami for the past 2 months. You are highly suspicious of tuberculosis. His sputum smear x 3 is negative for AFB.

Which of the following is more likely to be diagnostic for tuberculosis?

A. Repeat sputums
B. Acid-fast smear of pleural fluid
C. Pleural biopsy
D. CT scan of the chest
E. ACE levels

74.

A 56-year-old male is brought to your office because his wife complains of his constant snoring. She reports that he seems to stop breathing sometimes at night. He does report unrefreshed sleep, headaches upon awakening, and takes a nap nearly every day in his office after lunch. You suspect obstructive sleep apnea and order a polysomnogram. The report indicates that the patient has an AHI (apnea/hypopnea index) of 18 events/hour associated with oxygen desaturations as low as 79%.

Which of the following is true about obstructive sleep apnea (OSA)?

    A. Patients with treated OSA have a higher incidence of hypertension.
    B. Nocturnal oxygen alone has been shown to be an effective therapy.
    C. Neck circumference < 16 inches is a risk factor for OSA.
    D. CPAP (continuous positive airway pressure) can be effective in eliminating all respiratory related events due to OSA.
    E. Treatment with CPAP has not been shown to reduce subsequent cardiovascular events in patients with coronary artery disease.

75.

A 32-year-old female comes to your office to establish primary care. Her past medical history is only notable for asthma, diagnosed as a teenager. She reports symptoms nearly daily that can range from dry cough, worse at night, and exertional dyspnea. She denies any symptoms consistent with reflux disease but does endorse occasional chest tightness and burning, particularly when she tries to jog outside in the morning. She smokes 1/2 ppd and has been doing so for 11 years. She denies any pets. Family history is notable for a brother with asthma. Her medications include theophylline, salmeterol inhaler once daily, and albuterol nebulizer three times a day.

Which of the following regarding asthma is true?

    A. Inhaled corticosteroids should be considered only in patients with persistent asthma who have severe nocturnal symptoms.
    B. Prior to exercise or during periods of acute shortness of breath, long-acting beta-agonists should be used.
    C. Proton pump inhibitors are helpful in asthma control if a patient has asymptomatic GERD.
    D. Patients may have pulmonary function tests that are normal.
    E. A negative methacholine challenge test does not rule out the diagnosis of asthma.

76.

A 57-year-old male presents with a 14-month history of progressive dyspnea associated with exertion. It is associated with a dry cough with no specific triggers. He denies fever, chills, chest pain, or other constitutional symptoms. He is a lifelong non-smoker and has no specific medical history. He takes no medications and spent the majority of his life working as a management consultant in an office-based setting. On examination, he is thin, slightly tachypneic but without respiratory distress. His oxygen saturation at rest is 92% but declines to 86% with exertion after three minutes. On examination, he has digital clubbing but no cyanosis or edema. His lung exam reveals dry, coarse inspiratory crackles without wheezing. Remainder of the exam is unremarkable. Chest CT is interpreted as the following: "there are extensive bibasilar areas of fibrotic lung changes with honeycombing, traction bronchiectasis, and subpleural blebs. There are no areas of ground glass opacification. This is most consistent with a picture radiographically of pulmonary fibrosis."

Which of the following is true regarding idiopathic pulmonary fibrosis (IPF)?

A. Clubbing is commonly seen.
B. It is associated with a restrictive pattern on pulmonary function tests.
C. Surgical biopsy is not required to make diagnosis.
D. There is no specific pharmacologic treatment regimen that has been proven to improve survival in patients with IPF.
E. All of the answer options are true.

77.

A 19-year-old male presents to the local college infirmary with complaints of fever, cough, and chest pain. A review of his chart indicates the patient was seen for sore throat approximately 2 weeks prior to onset of current illness.

Which of the following is his most likely diagnosis?

A. *Streptococcus pyogenes*
B. *Klebsiella pneumoniae*
C. *Legionella*
D. *Chlamydophila* (formerly known as *Chlamydia*) *pneumoniae*

78.

A 20-year-old woman comes to the office for her routine checkup. She has a past history of asthma and presently is being treated with albuterol MDI on prn basis. She states she uses the inhaler at least once a day for wheezing. She admits to awakening from sleep 3–4 times per week for cough/wheeze. Past History: Hospitalized 1–2 times/year, ER visits approx. 6 times/year, 2 prior ICU admits at ages 6 and 8. Previously treated with inhaled steroids for 4–6 weeks around the time of hospital discharge (noticed no benefit). Requires oral steroid bursts every 6–8 weeks for 3–5 days.

PE: Essentially normal
Office Spirometry: FVC 88%, FEV_1 59%, FEF_{25-75} 48%

Based on the guidelines, how would this patient be classified?

A. Mild intermittent
B. Mild persistent
C. Moderate persistent
D. Severe persistent

79.

A 17-year-old woman presents to your office with fever for 3 days up to 105° F, complaints of severe sore throat, refusal to swallow, and is speaking with a "hot potato" voice. On exam her oropharynx is erythematous with exudates, and the uvula is displaced laterally.

Which of the following is the most likely etiology?

A. Retropharyngeal abscess
B. Acute pharyngitis
C. Peritonsillar abscess
D. Epiglottitis

80.

A 25-year-old woman with past history of mild persistent asthma presents with exacerbation of asthma. This is the fourth exacerbation in 3 months. Prior to 3 months ago, she had been well controlled with last exacerbation being at age 6. On presentation today she had increased cough productive of brown sputum (described as plugs) and wheezing. With each exacerbation a CXR was obtained showing infiltrates in different areas, usually upper lobes. Lab evaluation showed elevated peripheral blood eosinophil count.

Which of the following is her most likely etiology?

A. GE reflux
B. Chronic sinusitis
C. Allergic bronchopulmonary aspergillosis
D. Aspiration pneumonia

81.

A 65-year-old man presents with fever, chills, cough, and dyspnea for 3 days duration. This is associated with right-sided pleuritic chest pain as well as fatigue and mild nausea. His past medical history is only notable for hypertension for which he takes a thiazide diuretic. He has a 15-pack/year history of smoking but quit 10 years ago. On physical exam, his vitals are: T 102.4° F, RR 24, BP 100/45, O_2 sat 92%. Lung exam reveals dullness to percussion with diminished breath sounds from mid-right lung to base. The remainder of the exam is not pertinent. PA/Lat and decubitus chest radiograph films reveal a free flowing moderate-size pleural effusion. Thoracentesis is performed using ultrasound guidance and sent for multiple studies.

Which one of the following findings on pleural fluid studies would necessitate complete pleural fluid drainage with tube thoracostomy?

A. LDH level of 100
B. Pleural fluid protein/serum protein ratio less than 0.5
C. Growth of *Streptococcus pneumoniae*
D. Pleural pH = 7.42
E. White blood cell count of 5,000

82.

A 27-year-old young woman came to the Emergency Department complaining of pleuritic chest pain of several hours duration. She was not a smoker but gave a history of using birth control pills. Her chest x-ray and physical exam were normal except for splinting with deep inspirations. Arterial blood gas showed pH 7.45, $PaCO_2$ 31 mmHg, HCO_3 21 mEq/L, PaO_2 83 mmHg (breathing ambient air; PB 747 mmHg).

What should be the next step in management?

A. Discharge with pain medication
B. Consider SSRI for panic attacks
C. Diagnostic imaging to exclude pulmonary embolus
D. Start bicarbonate infusion
E. Start PO fluoroquinolone for treatment of pneumonia

83.

A 33-year-old woman presents with facial pain and nasal congestion. She reports she had the onset of sore throat and rhinorrhea 5 days ago. Over the past 48 hours she has had facial pressure over the maxillary sinus and yellow nasal discharge. On exam, T 99.2° F, P 90, BP 110/70. Nose: swollen turbinates. Neck: no adenopathy. Chest: clear

Which of the following treatments would you recommend?

A. Decongestants/nasal irrigation
B. Decongestants/nasal irrigation + Amoxicillin
C. Decongestants/nasal irrigation + TMP/Sulfa
D. Decongestants/nasal irrigation + Amoxicillin-clavulanate
E. Decongestants/nasal irrigation + Metronidazole

84.

A 68-year-old woman is admitted to a nursing home, and one year later she develops a cough. Workup is implemented and she has a positive PPD. A CXR is done and shows a left apical infiltrate, and sputums are positive for acid-fast organisms. She is placed in immediate respiratory isolation.

Which of the following do you recommend for your patient?

A. Further TB workup is necessary to determine what should be done.
B. Start INH only.
C. Start INH, rifampin, PZA, and ethambutol.
D. Start INH and rifampin.
E. Await sensitivities to begin therapy.

85.

On the Boards, sometimes it can be helpful to look where the disease is occurring in the lungs.

Which of the following interstitial lung diseases has upper lobe predominance?

A. Rheumatoid fibrosis
B. Pulmonary infiltrates related to scleroderma
C. Lymphangitic carcinomatosis
D. Silicosis
E. Asbestosis

86.

A 26-year-old woman presents with complaints of shortness of breath. She states that she first noticed the shortness of breath about 5 months ago. It mainly occurs when she is exercising, and she is unable to jog anymore because of shortness of breath. Recently she has been awakened at night with shortness of breath and has the feeling that she can't catch her breath. She has not had any fever, cough, or sputum production. She denies orthopnea.

Her physical examination is significant for the following:

Heart:	RRR without murmurs, rubs, or gallops
Lungs:	Clear to auscultation
Abdomen:	Benign
Extremities:	No edema, clubbing, or cyanosis

CXR is normal.
Office spirometry is normal for age.
ABG on room air: pH 7.40, $PaCO_2$, 42 mmHg, and PaO_2 of 93 mmHg

Which of the following diagnostic tests would you perform next?

    A. Flow-volume loop
    B. Echocardiography
    C. Full pulmonary function tests with diffusing capacity determination
    D. Bronchoprovocation (methacholine challenge test)
    E. High-resolution CT of the chest

87.

You are presented a patient with asthma exacerbation. He is on beta-blocker medications after a recent myocardial infarction.

Which of the following agents would be useful in an acute exacerbation to improve bronchodilation quickly?

    A. Ipratropium
    B. Cromolyn sodium
    C. Epinephrine
    D. Albuterol
    E. Prednisone

88.

A 50-year-old school teacher presents with concerns about asbestos exposure. He has been in a school that has recently been closed because of concerns of asbestos.

Which of the following manifestations of asbestos-induced lung disease has the shortest latency period of occurrence?

A. Asbestosis
B. Benign asbestos pleural effusions
C. Diffuse pleural effusions
D. Localized pleural effusions
E. Mesothelioma

89.

Which of the following is associated with lower lobe interstitial infiltrates?

A. Ankylosing spondylitis
B. Eosinophilic granuloma
C. Silicosis
D. Rheumatoid fibrosis
E. *Pneumocystis jiroveci* pneumonia in patients on inhaled pentamidine therapy

90.

A 45-year-old non-smoker presents with dyspnea on exertion for 2 months. He has bibasilar crackles and has restrictive disease on pulmonary function testing. He is sent for transbronchial biopsy. On further questioning you learn he works with beryllium.

Which of the following would help differentiate between sarcoid and berylliosis?

A. Non-caseating granulomas on biopsy
B. Kveim skin test
C. ACE level
D. Lymphocyte transformation test (LTT) on BAL lymphocytes and/or blood
E. CD4 to CD8 ratios

91.

A 65-year-old man presents with progressive dyspnea on exertion associated with a dry cough. This has been occurring for over two years. He has a 25 pack-year history of smoking. Occupational history includes over 30 years working in a factory that manufactured glass bowls and vases as well as 2 years working in an auto body shop doing brake repair jobs. His chest radiograph is described as: "bilateral apical regions of parenchymal fibrosis with coalescent areas of consolidation." Previous testing indicates an FEV_1/FVC ratio of 80%, FEV_1 that is 1.5 L (56% predicted) and a TLC of 3.50 L (50% predicted).

Which of the following occupational causes of interstitial lung disease is associated with a higher risk of tuberculosis?

A. Coal worker's pneumoconiosis
B. Berylliosis
C. Silicosis
D. Asbestosis
E. Byssinosis

92.

Which of the following is true regarding pulmonary emboli?

A. The most specific ECG change is tachycardia.
B. CXR will usually show an infiltrate distal to the embolus.
C. A normal venogram of the lower extremities rules out pulmonary embolism.
D. All pulmonary emboli originate in the lower extremities.
E. The hypoxia associated with a large pulmonary embolus is due to a right-to-left shunt caused by perfusion of poorly ventilated areas.

93.

A 32-year-old female complains of cough for 1 year duration. She also has exertional dyspnea as well as a purplish-colored rash that recurs intermittently across her cheeks and shins. Chest radiograph reveals bilateral hilar lymphadenopathy. She has no significant past medical history, no significant family history, and currently works in a supermarket. She denies smoking, alcohol, or drug use except for occasional marijuana. Mediastinoscopy is done to assess the enlarged lymph nodes. Biopsy indicates "the presence of well-formed non-caseating granulomas." Bacterial, AFB, and fungal cultures are all negative.

Which of the following disorders is the most likely diagnosis?

A. Tuberculosis
B. Berylliosis
C. Lymphoma
D. Histoplasmosis
E. Sarcoidosis

94.

You are presented with an HIV-infected patient with possible tuberculosis versus atypical mycobacterium lung infection.

Which of the following would make you lean more toward tuberculosis as an etiology?

A. HIV for 20 years
B. CD4 of 450
C. CD4 of 20
D. Taking trimethoprim/sulfamethoxazole for prophylaxis
E. Acid fast smears of the sputum are negative

95.

A 40-year-old nurse presents with a PPD of 15 mm. A CXR reveals a cavitary lesion. Initial sputum reveals acid-fast organisms with cultures pending. She works and lives in rural Iowa where resistant tuberculosis has not been documented.

Which of the following do you recommend for her?

A. INH alone is sufficient therapy.
B. Do not start therapy until the cultures return with sensitivities.
C. Begin 4-drug therapy with INH, RIF, PZA, and ethambutol.
D. Begin 5-drug therapy with INH, RIF, PZA, ethambutol, and streptomycin.
E. Because the risk of resistance is low, INH and RIF only are sufficient therapy.

96.

A 29-year-old female is 32 weeks pregnant with her first pregnancy. She has a history of mild intermittent asthma for which she uses an albuterol inhaler occasionally. She presents to your office with a 5-day history of increased dyspnea associated with dry cough and some intermittent wheezing. She denies any reflux symptoms, fever, nasal drainage, or recent sick contacts. On exam, she is slightly tachypneic with a respiratory rate of 20; the remainder of the vital signs are normal. Lung exam reveals mild expiratory wheezing with slightly prolonged expiratory phase.

Which of the following is true regarding asthma in pregnancy?

A. Controlled asthma during pregnancy is associated with a higher risk of preeclampsia.
B. Budesonide is the only inhaled steroid with a Class X rating in regard to safety in pregnancy.
C. The management principles for asthma are the same in pregnant and non-pregnant patients.
D. Oral corticosteroids would be contraindicated in patients with asthma exacerbation and pregnancy.
E. Approximately 80% of patients with asthma will have symptoms that worsen with pregnancy.

97.

A 56-year-old male was diagnosed with gastric cancer approximately 5 months ago. He has been initiated on chemotherapy. He presents to the Emergency Department with acute onset of right-sided chest pain that is worse with inspiration. This is associated with significant dyspnea on rest and exertion. He has noted some mild left lower extremity edema with associated erythema. His vitals are as follows: heart rate 125 bpm, RR 28, blood pressure 120/75, oxygen saturations of 92% on room air. Arterial blood gas reveals: pH 7.33, pCO_2 33, PaO_2 65. He appears anxious and slightly dyspneic without any accessory muscle use. He does have 2+ edema of the left lower extremity from the mid thigh distally to the dorsum of the foot. There is no pain with palpation of the calf. Pulmonary embolus is suspected and a chest CT angiogram is performed and is shown below. Troponin is ordered and is 8x the normal value. Bedside echocardiogram reveals a poorly contractile right ventricle that is enlarged, tricuspid regurgitation with pulmonary hypertension, and bowing of the interventricular septum toward the left ventricle. The patient has no known risk factors for bleeding.

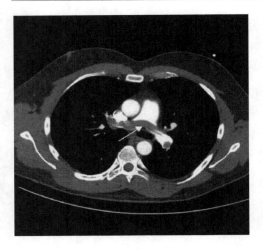

Which of the following interventions would provide a survival benefit for this patient?

   A. Initiation of anti-coagulation with low-molecular-weight heparin
   B. Placement of inferior vena caval filter
   C. Infusion of 100 mg of tissue plasminogen activator (tPA)
   D. Placement of right heart catheter to assess pulmonary arterial pressures

98.

What is the most likely fungal lung disease in a patient from Arkansas or Missouri with a draining leg lesion?

   A. Histoplasmosis
   B. Blastomycosis
   C. Aspergillosis
   D. Coccidioidomycosis
   E. *Streptococcus pneumoniae*

99.

An 18-year-old female with a history of poorly controlled asthma presents to the Emergency Department with a 3-day history of worsening shortness of breath. Upon presentation, she is in marked respiratory distress with accessory muscle use, a respiratory rate of 40 breaths/minute, and very poor air movement. She initially was alert but has become increasingly lethargic. Chest radiograph was unremarkable. The decision is made to intubate the patient and place on invasive mechanical ventilation due to respiratory failure. Post intubation radiograph reveals appropriate placement of the endotracheal tube without any other changes. The patient is started on intravenous steroids and continuous nebulization of albuterol. Her ventilator settings are as follows:

Respiratory rate: 16, Tidal Volume: 400 mL, FiO_2: 50%, PEEP 5. The patient is heavily sedated and has no spontaneous respiratory rate.

After 1 hour, arterial blood gas is as follows:

pH: 7.22, pCO_2: 60, PO_2 130, HCO_3 23.

Peak inspiratory pressure is 42 cm. There is no significant intrinsic PEEP.

Which of the following is the most appropriate next step in the management of this patient?

A. Increase the respiratory rate on the ventilator to 22 breaths per minute
B. Increase the FiO_2 to 60%
C. Increase the PEEP to 10 cm H_2O
D. Administer 100 mEq of sodium bicarbonate
E. Decrease the tidal volume to 300 mL

100.

Which of the following is the treatment for acute methemoglobinemia?

A. Sodium pentathlon
B. 100% oxygen and methylene blue
C. Carbon monoxide and methylene blue
D. Ascorbic acid
E. Carbon dioxide and methylene blue

101.

Which of the following values is consistent with emphysema?

	%TLC	%DLCO
A.	Normal	Normal
B.	Low	Low
C.	High	Low
D.	Low	Normal
E.	Low	High

102.

An asthmatic presents in respiratory distress. He requires mechanical ventilation.

Which of the following parameters is best for an asthmatic?

	Rate	Tidal Volume	Flows
A.	High	High	High
B.	High	Low	Low
C.	Low	High	Low
D.	Low	Low	High
E.	Low	High	High

103.

A 30-year-old non-smoker presents with worsening shortness of breath. A CXR is done and shows emphysematous bullae in the bases consistent with early-onset COPD.

Which of the following is a likely etiology for his condition?

A. AIDS
B. Berylliosis
C. Sarcoidosis
D. Homozygous α_1-antitrypsin deficiency
E. Eosinophilic granuloma

104.

What do "egg-shell" calcifications make you think of?

A. Histoplasmosis
B. Blastomycosis
C. Silicosis
D. Sarcoidosis
E. Asbestosis

105.

What is eosinophilic granulomatosis in association with lytic bone lesions, diabetes insipidus, and exophthalmus called?

A. Treacher-Collins syndrome
B. Hannaman-Cross syndrome
C. Hand-Schüller-Christian syndrome
D. Maple-syrup lung disease
E. Löffler syndrome

106.

A 65-year-old man presents to his physician's office with a 9-month history of dyspnea on exertion associated with a mild cough. He has daily sputum expectoration, most pronounced in the morning. He has a past medical history notable for coronary artery disease for which he is on aspirin, simvastatin, and atenolol. He is a 50 pack-year smoker and works in an office-based setting. On physical exam, he has no evidence of resting or exertional hypoxemia. His breath sounds are moderately-to-severely diminished without any adventitial sounds. Pulmonary function tests reveal: forced expiratory volume in 1 second (FEV_1) is 1.5 L (60% of predicted), forced vital capacity (FVC) is 2.3 L, and the FEV_1/FVC ratio is 0.65. TLC is 5.25 L (125% predicted) and DLCO is 25 mmHg (56% predicted).

Which of the following will be most effective for improving this patient's long-term survival?

A. Inhaled corticosteroids combined with long-acting beta-agonists
B. Oxygen therapy
C. Inhaled tiotropium
D. Pulmonary rehabilitation
E. Smoking cessation

107.

On the Board exam they will frequently give you scenarios in which a patient will present with shortness of breath and you have to discern the etiology. Some of their favorites include high-risk procedures/conditions for pulmonary embolism.

If prophylaxis is not given, which of the following patients is considered at <u>highest</u> risk for pulmonary embolism?

A. A 30-year-old man undergoing tonsillectomy
B. A 90-year-old man undergoing cataract surgery
C. A 50-year-old man undergoing knee replacement
D. A 35-year-old woman undergoing hysterectomy
E. A 50-year-old woman undergoing hysterectomy

108.

A 40-year-old distance runner presents with a new diagnosis of lymphoma. She has been doing well but presents with new onset pleural effusion. A pleural tap is done and shows white-appearing exudative fluid.

Which of the following is causing the fluid to be white?

A. The calcium level of the fluid is > 10 mg/dL, and there are calcium globules causing the whitish color.
B. The triglyceride level of the fluid is > 115 mg/dL, and there are chylomicrons causing the whitish color.
C. The WBC of the fluid is > 1,000, and there are clumped WBCs causing the whitish color.
D. The rheumatoid factor of the fluid is high, and the RF causes a whitish color.
E. The triglyceride level of the fluid is < 50 mg/dL, and cholesterol causes the whitish color.

109.

A 77-year-old man presents to the Emergency Department with a 5-day history of increased dyspnea above his baseline, productive cough, fever to 102.1° F, and foul smelling sputum. In addition, he says he always has dyspnea when lying down, but this has become more pronounced over the last 3 weeks. He has chronic lower extremity edema for which he takes a "fluid pill." On review of his previous hospital record, he is noted to have an echocardiogram report from one year prior with a left ventricular ejection fraction of 25%. A chest radiograph is obtained and shows a left-sided infiltrate and moderate-size effusion. He is initiated on antibiotics for coverage of community-acquired pneumonia.

Which of the following tests would be most helpful to determine if the effusion is due to congestive heart failure versus related to pneumonia?

A. LDH
B. Cell count with differential
C. Adenosine deaminase
D. Glucose
E. Triglycerides

110.

For which of the following is a 5 mm PPD considered significant?

A. Health-care workers
B. IV drug abusers
C. Prisoners
D. Homeless persons
E. Close contact with a documented case

CARDIOLOGY

111.

A 35-year-old woman presents to your office with chest pain for the past six months. She describes the pain as a non-radiating substernal pressure sensation, lasting from a few minutes to as long as four hours. She does not get the pain while walking her dog around a local soccer field every evening, but she occasionally has it when lying down at night. It has been occurring more frequently over the past four weeks. Her only other medical problems are moderate obesity and hypertension. She does not smoke and is not taking oral contraceptives. She is not aware of her cholesterol level, but she remembers being told that her blood sugar was previously normal. Her family history is unremarkable.

On physical examination, her blood pressure was 140/90 mmHg and heart rate was 85. Other than obesity, the examination was normal. A complete blood count and chemistry panel were normal except for a cholesterol level of 220 mg/dL. An electrocardiogram showed normal sinus rhythm and nonspecific ST and T wave changes.

Which of the following statements is true regarding this patient?

A. She has about a 10% chance of having a significant stenosis in at least one coronary artery.
B. Standard exercise stress testing will have a high degree of accuracy in determining if she has coronary artery disease.
C. If she has 2 mm of upsloping ST segment depression during a standard exercise stress test, she is extremely likely to have significant coronary disease.
D. An immediate post exercise and four-hour recovery nuclear imaging study with thallium^{201} will not improve the accuracy of a standard exercise stress test in this patient.
E. An exercise capacity of 10 METs will risk stratify this patient to a 10% five-year cardiac mortality.

112.

A patient with a systolic murmur is found to have aortic stenosis by echocardiography. The velocity of flow across the aortic valve is determined by Doppler analysis to be 4 m/sec.

What is the peak systolic gradient across this valve?

A. 16 mmHg
B. 24 mmHg
C. 44 mmHg
D. 64 mmHg
E. 96 mmHg

113.

A 63-year-old man with a history of classical angina for the past three years reports a gradual increase in the frequency of the pain and a decrease in the amount of effort required to cause it. His medications include aspirin, metoprolol, and simvastatin. You obtain a standard exercise stress, during which he exercises for 4 METs. You stop the exercise test at that time because of a drop in systolic blood pressure from 120 to 90 mmHg. He did not have chest pain at this level of exertion. Electrocardiograms obtained at rest and at 4 METs of exercise are presented:

Resting ECG

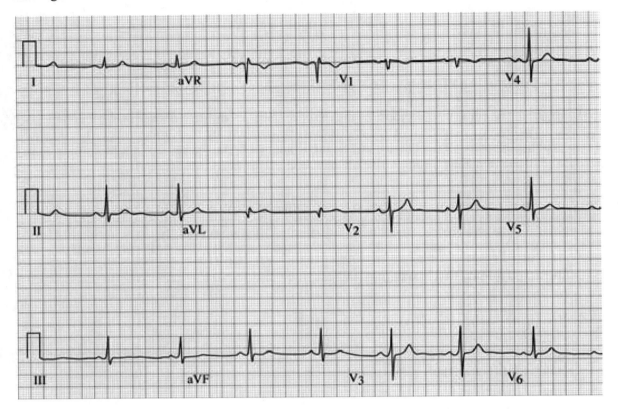

ECG at 4 METs of exercise

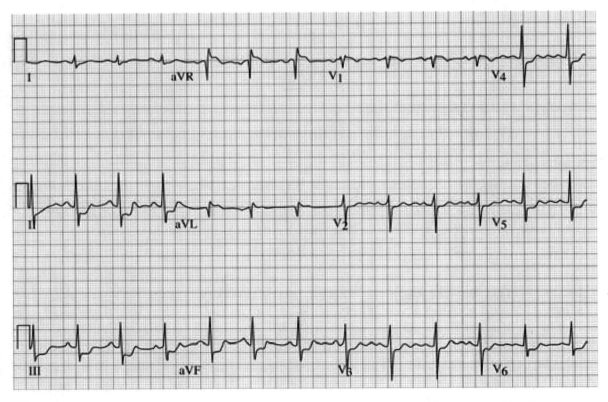

Which of the following statements is true?

A. This patient has a 75% chance of having significant coronary disease.
B. The exercise stress test should be repeated with a thallium imaging study for greater accuracy.
C. He should have coronary angiography as soon as possible.
D. He should have medical therapy alone, with the addition of a nitroglycerin patch and an increase in the dose of metoprolol.
E. He should be referred for consultation with a gastroenterologist.

114.

A 75-year-old woman with a history of a previous myocardial infarction comes to the Emergency Department complaining of three episodes of syncope in the past 24 hours. She has had slowly increasing dyspnea over the past 3 weeks, and now has to sleep propped up on 3 pillows. Physical examination demonstrates an apical third heart sound. Her initial ECG is shown:

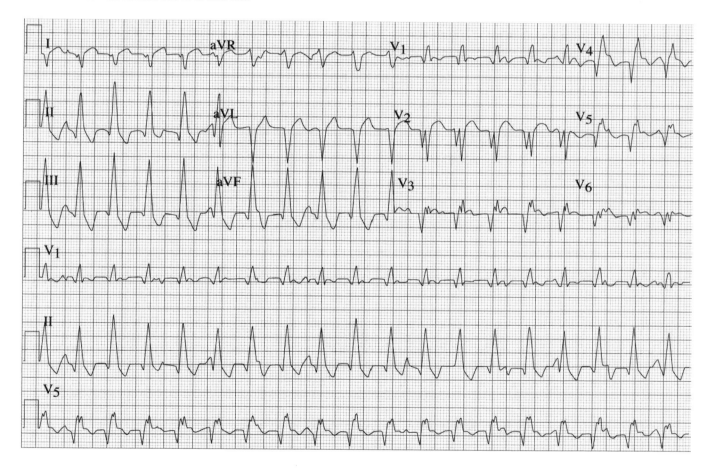

An examination of this patient's neck veins is most likely to show which of the following?

A. A rapid *x* and *y* descent
B. Irregular cannon *a* waves and large *v* waves
C. A positive Kussmaul's sign
D. Regular large *a* waves and small *v* waves
E. Engorged neck veins without pulsations

115.

All of the following right heart sounds become louder on inspiration <u>except</u> which of the following:

    A. Pulmonic regurgitation murmur
    B. Tricuspid regurgitation murmur
    C. Right-sided third heart sound
    D. Tricuspid stenosis murmur
    E. Pulmonic ejection sound

116.

A 43-year-old woman comes to your office complaining of 6 months of increasing dyspnea. Recently she has had to stop virtually all activities except moving about the house. In the course of her evaluation, an echocardiogram demonstrates a greatly enlarged right atrium and right ventricle with a pulmonary artery systolic pressure of 95 mmHg. The left heart has normal size and function. She is eventually diagnosed as having primary pulmonary hypertension.

Which of the following would you expect to hear on auscultation of her second heart sound?

    A. A soft P_2
    B. A widely split second heart sound
    C. A single second heart sound
    D. Paradoxical splitting of the second heart sound
    E. A fixed split of the second heart sound

117.

A 45-year-old woman comes to your Emergency Department with a complaint of 2 hours of severe anterior chest pain. She has no history of cardiac disease. She describes a sharp, stabbing pain that radiates to her left arm and neck, worsened somewhat by respiration. She also has moderate dyspnea. Her cardiac risk factors include current smoking and hypertension. On physical examination, her heart rate is 95 and blood pressure 165/110 mmHg. The remainder of the examination is normal. Her laboratory data is all normal except a white blood count of 11.6 x 10^9/L. Cardiac markers are negative. A chest x-ray is normal. Her electrocardiogram follows:

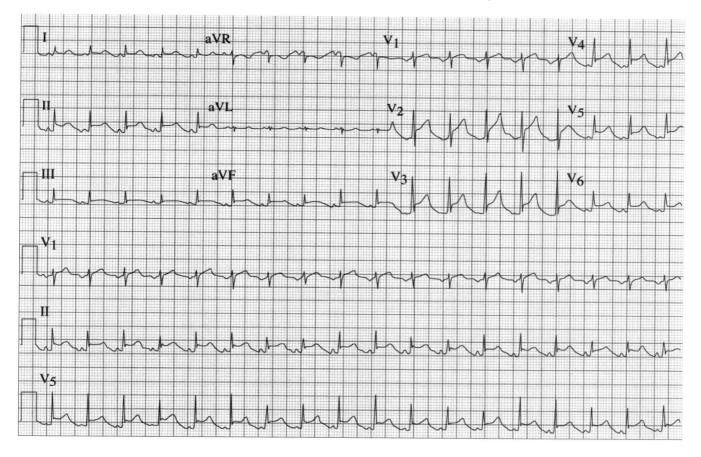

Which of the following statements is true?

A. This patient should be transferred immediately to a tertiary care center for percutaneous coronary intervention.
B. Fibrinolytic therapy with intravenous tissue plasminogen activator is indicated.
C. An echocardiogram is likely to show a segmental wall motion abnormality of the left ventricle.
D. Treatment with a nonsteroidal antiinflammatory agent is indicated.
E. Abdominojugular reflux is usually present in this condition.

118.

A 68-year-old man comes to the Emergency Department complaining of 12 hours of substernal chest pain, nausea, mild dyspnea, and lightheadedness. He has no previous history of cardiac disease. His cardiac risk factors include age, male sex, diabetes, and current cigarette smoking. On examination, his heart rate is 70 and his blood pressure is 120/75 mmHg. He has irregular cannon *a* waves in the jugular venous pulse. His lungs have a few bibasilar crackles. He has a soft apical third heart sound on auscultation. His initial electrocardiogram appears below.

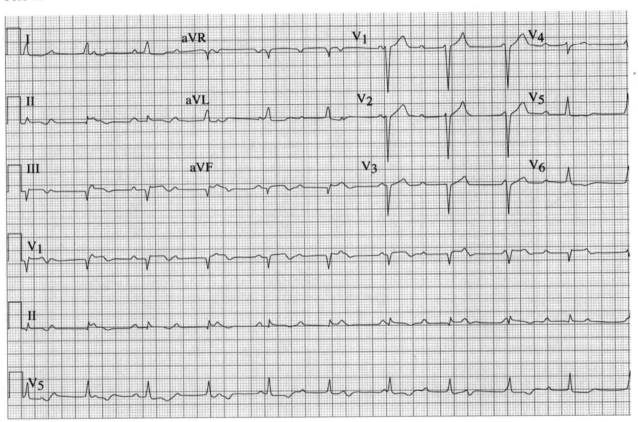

Which of the following statements is true?

A. Fibrinolytic therapy is likely to substantially decrease his in-hospital and 30-day mortality.
B. He is likely to require a permanent transvenous pacemaker.
C. Temporary transvenous pacing is not necessary at this time because of the normal heart rate and blood pressure.
D. A radionuclide ventriculogram (MUGA) showing a left ventricular ejection fraction of 30% would be an indication for coronary angiography.
E. Prognosis in this patient's condition is excellent (cardiac mortality less than 5% at one year).

119.

A 56-year-old man comes to the Emergency Department complaining of six hours of constant dull substernal chest pain. He has had chest pain intermittently for the past year but has not sought medical attention. He has an episode of pain 2–3 times per week, occurring at rest and with exercise, and sometimes at night. The pain lasts from 20 minutes to several hours. He regularly cares for his three horses, lifting 100-pound bales of hay and raking out their stalls, and this activity is infrequently associated with chest pain. His cardiac risk factors include age, male sex, and a strong family history of early coronary disease. In fact, he sought medical attention on this occasion because his 43-year-old brother had a heart attack in the previous week. His physical examination is unremarkable. Initial cardiac markers are negative, and his electrocardiogram is normal.

Which of the following statements is true?

   A. He has a noncardiac cause of chest pain and should be discharged from the Emergency Department and a follow-up appointment with his primary care provider should be arranged.
   B. He should be given a prescription for a beta-blocker and sublingual nitroglycerin and a follow-up appointment with his primary care provider should be arranged.
   C. He should be observed for at least 12 hours after symptom onset and additional cardiac markers and electrocardiogram should be obtained.
   D. He should be admitted to the hospital and started on aspirin, clopidogrel, and a low-molecular weight heparin.
   E. He should have early cardiac catheterization and probably coronary intervention.

120.

A 67-year-old woman presents with 4 hours of substernal chest pain. An electrocardiogram shows ST segment elevation in leads V1–V5. She has no contraindications to fibrinolytic therapy.

Which of the following statements is true?

   A. This is a higher risk presentation than if she had had a new LBBB on her electrocardiogram.
   B. Streptokinase plus heparin has been shown to have a more favorable effect on mortality than other fibrinolytic agents.
   C. The combination of streptokinase, tissue plasminogen activator (tPA), and heparin has been shown to have a more favorable effect on mortality than other fibrinolytic agents.
   D. Subcutaneous heparin has been shown to be just as effective in decreasing mortality as intravenous heparin.
   E. The combination of tPA and intravenous heparin has been shown to have a more favorable effect on mortality than other fibrinolytic agents.

121.

A 72-year-old man presents with 3 hours of chest pain radiating down his left arm. He also has moderate dyspnea. He has a history of known coronary artery disease with coronary bypass graft surgery 5 years ago. His physical examination shows a heart rate of 85, a blood pressure of 145/95 mmHg, and moderate elevation of the jugular venous pressure. His first troponin I level is 13.6 ng/mL. An electrocardiogram shows ST segment depression in the lateral leads.

Which of the following statements is true?

A. This patient is at high risk and should receive immediate fibrinolytic therapy with tPA and intravenous unfractionated heparin.
B. He should receive aspirin, clopidogrel, a low-molecular-weight heparin (or some other type of antithrombin therapy), and possibly a GP IIb/IIIa antagonist.
C. Beta-blockers should be avoided because of his heart failure.
D. A stress study should be performed prior to discharge to determine if coronary angiography is necessary.
E. Clopidogrel should be continued for only 1 week.

122.

An 85-year-old woman was brought to the Emergency Department because of increasing confusion. Her son is able to tell you that she has some kind of "heart problem" and gives you a list of her medications, which include digoxin, amlodipine, and furosemide. She has a history of hypertension. On examination, her heart rate is 80 and blood pressure 170/110. She has some crackles in both lung bases. She is moderately confused and combative, which her son says is new for her. She has no focal neurological defects. Her initial troponin I is 55 ng/mL. Serum digoxin level is 1.1 ng/dL. A chest x-ray shows cardiomegaly and pulmonary vascular congestion. Her electrocardiogram is shown below.

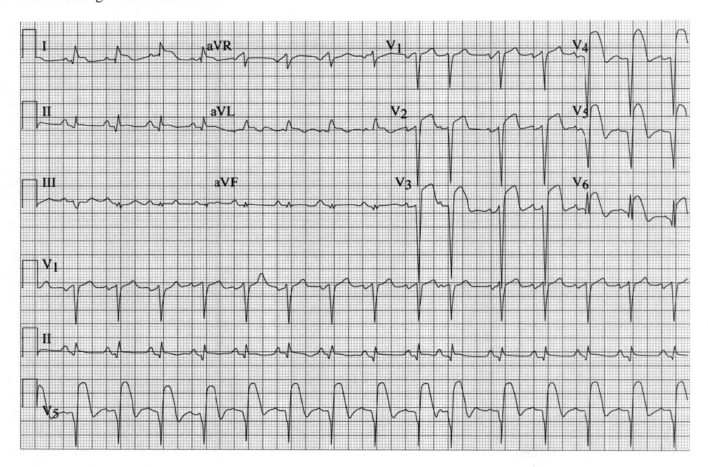

Her oxygen saturation on room air is 55%.

You begin therapy with oxygen, furosemide, aspirin, heparin, cautious administration of an angiotensin converting enzyme inhibitor, and carvedilol. She slowly improves over the next 3 days and becomes less confused. On the fourth day, while sitting on the bedside commode, she has a syncopal episode and falls to the floor. She is immediately noted to be unconscious and to have labored respirations and a weak, thready pulse. Her rhythm on the bedside monitor is sinus tachycardia.

She is intubated and ventilated and 500 mL of intravenous saline is administered. A stat echocardiogram is obtained.

Which one of the following is the echo most likely to demonstrate?

A. A large pericardial effusion with collapse of the right atrium and ventricle
B. A ventricular septal defect
C. Rupture of the posterior papillary muscle of the mitral valve and severe mitral regurgitation
D. Severe left ventricular systolic dysfunction with an estimated left ventricular ejection fraction of 10%
E. Severe aortic stenosis

123.

A 22-year-old woman who is in the third trimester of an otherwise unremarkable pregnancy presented to her obstetrician with the sudden onset of severe intrascapular pain and moderate dyspnea. On physical examination, she was reported to be exceedingly uncomfortable and could not remain still. Her heart rate was 110 and blood pressure 165/110 mmHg in the left arm. The office nurse cannot obtain a blood pressure reading in the right arm. She was hospitalized and you are consulted. On your examination, she has no pulses in the right arm and her right carotid pulse is weaker than the left. She also has a soft diastolic decrescendo murmur heard best at the lower left sternal border. Basic laboratory data is normal. An electrocardiogram shows sinus tachycardia.

Which of the following statements is true?

A. This patient is likely to have a DeBakey class III or a Stanford Type B dissection.
B. The drug of choice for this condition is intravenous nitroprusside alone.
C. An MRI of the chest is an appropriate diagnostic test for this condition.
D. An aortic dissection in this location can usually be treated conservatively.
E. An echocardiogram is not necessary.

124.

An 85-year-old man comes to your office complaining of several recent episodes of syncope. He says he usually has these when he tries to work around his house. His wife has observed two of these episodes, and she describes a sudden loss of consciousness lasting for 20–30 seconds. He does not lose bowel or bladder control and is alert and oriented upon awakening. He denies chest pain, palpitations, or dyspnea. He has had no prior cardiac complaints. His cardiac risk factors are age, male sex, and hypertension. On physical examination, his heart rate is 60 and his blood pressure 125/75 mmHg. His jugular venous pressure is normal. His carotid pulses are normal except for a faint transmitted murmur bilaterally. His first heart sound is normal, but the second heart sound is single. There is an apical fourth heart sound. There is a nearly holosystolic murmur heard loudest at the apex. His laboratory data is all normal.

His electrocardiogram is shown:

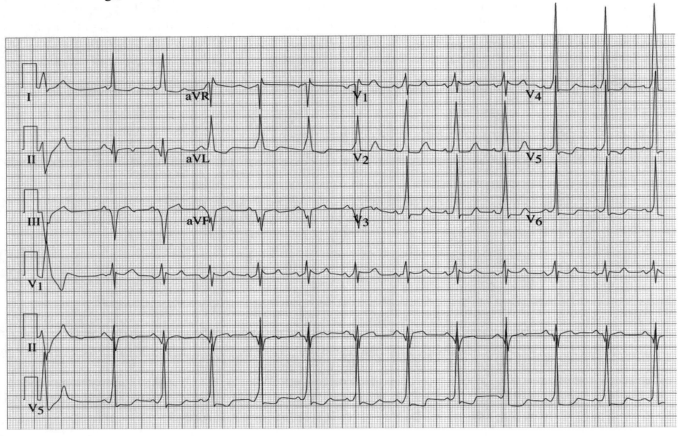

Which of the following statements is true?

    A. There is a risk of sudden death in this condition.
    B. The murmur would become louder upon standing or during the strain phase of the Valsalva maneuver.
    C. Treatment with afterload reduction therapy is indicated.
    D. Conservative therapy is indicated for this very elderly patient.
    E. If surgery were contemplated, an echocardiogram would provide sufficient information without having to have cardiac catheterization and coronary angiography.

125.

A 25-year-old woman in the third trimester of pregnancy comes to the Emergency Department after the sudden onset of severe dyspnea. She is tachypneic and her heart rate is 160. She is from Central America and has not sought prenatal care because of her immigrant status. Her electrocardiogram and chest x-ray are shown.

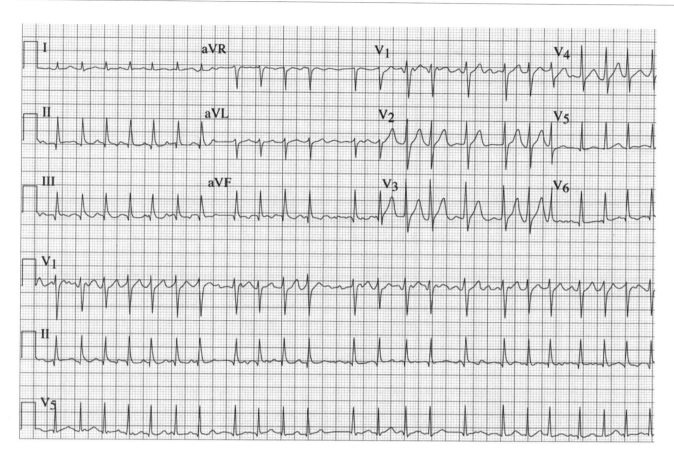

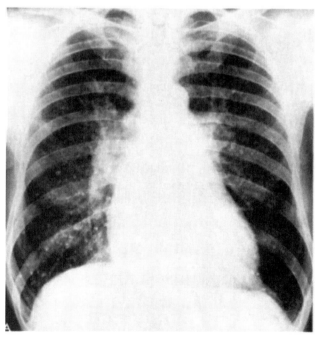

Which of the following statements is true?

    A. A pulmonic ejection sound is common in this condition.
    B. Sputum cultures for fungal infections are essential.
    C. Hemoptysis is a common feature of this condition, so patients should not be anticoagulated.
    D. Therapy with beta-blockers is contraindicated because of the heart failure seen on the chest x-ray.
    E. This abnormality develops earlier in patients from tropical countries.

126.

A 54-year-old man is enjoying himself at a local restaurant when he develops the sudden onset of severe dyspnea. He has no previous cardiac history and has been in good health otherwise. His wife drives him to your Emergency Department, whereupon he has a respiratory arrest and requires intubation and mechanical ventilation. On physical examination, his heart rate is 120 and his blood pressure is 85/50 mmHg. His neck veins are elevated to the angle of the jaw in the sitting position. His lungs have diffuse crackles and wheezes. There is a rapid heart rate without obvious extra sounds or murmurs. His extremities are cold and diaphoretic. Initial laboratory data shows normal CK and troponin levels. An electrocardiogram shows sinus tachycardia. A chest x-ray shows a normal-sized heart and gross pulmonary edema. An urgent echocardiogram is obtained, which shows severe mitral regurgitation.

Which of the following statements is true?

    A. This patient should have an immediate cardiothoracic surgical consultation.
    B. Blood cultures are likely to be positive, but that does not affect immediate management.
    C. If a murmur were to be heard in this patient, it would be holosystolic.
    D. Transient ischemia of the posterior papillary muscle is the most likely cause of this condition.
    E. This abnormality is more likely to occur in women.

127.

A 17-year-old Asian student is playing basketball when he collapses and becomes unresponsive. An initial examination by the trainer, who was at courtside, reveals that he is not breathing and does not have a palpable pulse. The school has a defibrillator at hand for all games, and 300 joules of energy are delivered to the student's chest. He recovers quickly and is immediately brought to your hospital and admitted to your coronary care unit. By the time you examine him, he is alert and his vital signs are stable. He has no previous history of heart disease or any other medical problem, and he denies illegal drug use. There is no history of sudden death in younger members of his family. His physical examination is entirely normal. Basic laboratory data show a normal complete blood count and chemistry panel. A chest x-ray shows moderate cardiomegaly. An electrocardiogram shows sinus rhythm with very large R waves in I, aVL, V5, and V6.

Which of the following statements is true?

    A. An echocardiogram will show asymmetric septal hypertrophy and a pressure gradient across the aortic outflow tract.
    B. Amiodarone has been shown to prolong survival in these patients.
    C. Atrial fibrillation is a frequent complication of this condition.
    D. Standing will produce a systolic murmur.
    E. The commonest cause of sudden death in this condition is associated with anomalous origin of a coronary artery.

128.

A 57-year-old man with advanced lung cancer presents with 24 hours of increasing dyspnea and pleuritic chest pain. He has no previous history of cardiac disease.

On examination, blood pressure is 85/40 mmHg and heart rate is 120 beats/minute. The neck veins are elevated above the clavicle in the sitting position. There are no murmurs or extra sounds. The breath sounds are decreased in the right base.

A right heart catheter is inserted from the right internal jugular vein, and the following pressures are obtained:

Location	Pressure (mmHg)
Right Atrium	21
Pulmonary Artery	45/20
Pulmonary Capillary Wedge	22

Which of the following is the correct diagnosis?

    A. Pulmonary embolism
    B. Acute myocardial infarction
    C. Constrictive pericarditis
    D. Cardiac tamponade
    E. Pneumonia

129.

A 77-year-old man with known ischemic heart disease and heart failure is admitted to your hospital with severe dyspnea. He reports that his baseline shortness of breath on climbing one flight of stairs has progressed over the past week to where he now has to sit sleeping upright in a chair. He denies chest pain or other symptoms. His other medical problems include diabetes and mild chronic renal failure. A previous echocardiogram showed segmental wall motion abnormalities of the left ventricle and an ejection fraction of 20%. On examination, his heart rate is 105 and blood pressure is 110/65 mmHg. His neck veins are elevated to the angle of the jaw in the sitting position. His lungs have diffuse crackles and wheezes throughout. He has a left parasternal lift, and the apical impulse is palpated to be 4 cm in diameter. There are left parasternal and apical third heart sounds, and a soft apical holosystolic murmur with radiation to the anterior axillary line. His laboratory is remarkable for a hemoglobin of 6.8 g/dL and an MCV of 68 fL, a BUN of 67 mg/dL, and a creatinine of 2.3 mg/dL, and a glucose level of 237 mg/dL. Cardiac markers, including CK and troponin I, are negative. A chest x-ray shows cardiomegaly, pulmonary edema, and bilateral pleural effusions. An electrocardiogram shows sinus tachycardia and an old extensive anterior myocardial infarction.

Which of the following statements is true?

    A. Obtaining a new echocardiogram is likely be extremely useful in managing this patient.
    B. The diameter of the apical impulse is consistent with left ventricular hypertrophy.
    C. This patient should have a cautious transfusion of packed red blood cells to bring his hemoglobin to above 10.
    D. Most patients with severe heart failure die of sudden cardiac death.
    E. There is no evidence of pulmonary hypertension in this patient.

130.

Which of the following statements regarding digoxin is true?

A. Digoxin has been shown to have an adverse effect on survival in patients with left ventricular ejection fractions less than 25%.
B. Toxic level of digoxin can be removed with hemodialysis.
C. The commonest arrhythmia produced by digoxin toxicity is atrial fibrillation.
D. The effectiveness of digoxin antibody therapy for digoxin toxicity should be assessed by subsequent serum digoxin levels.
E. Signs of digoxin toxicity may be present in a patient with serum levels in the therapeutic range.

131.

A 73-year-old man with Type 2 DM, CAD, HTN, and CHF presents with worsening symptoms of heart failure. He has had increased paroxysmal nocturnal dyspnea and orthopnea. He has had a 15-lb weight gain in the past month. On exam he has bilateral rales and 2+ pitting edema to the mid calf. Labs: HCT 32 (was 37 a month ago), Bun 20, Cr 1.1. Meds: glyburide, metformin, lisinopril, rosiglitazone, carvedilol, spironolactone, and nortriptyline.

What is the most likely cause of his increased CHF symptoms?

A. Metformin
B. Lisinopril
C. Spironolactone
D. Rosiglitazone
E. Carvedilol

132.

An 18-year-old woman is standing in line for college admission testing when she begins to feel lightheaded and falls to the ground. She is unresponsive. No seizure activity is noted. Her vital signs are stable. Though she looks somewhat pale, she regains consciousness within 3 minutes and within 15 minutes is back to her previous state. She says that she felt weak, and the room became "dark" to her just prior to "falling out." She says that she has not been ill and otherwise has had no medical problems. She does admit to frequently feeling lightheaded upon rising quickly from the supine or seated positions, and says that she may have passed out once before in church.

What is the most likely explanation for her syncopal episode?

A. Hypertrophic cardiomyopathy
B. Anomalous coronary artery
C. Long QT syndrome
D. Severe aortic stenosis
E. Neurocardiogenic (vasovagal) syncope

133.

A 63-year-old man with severe osteoarthritis of his hip is scheduled for elective left hip replacement in one week. During your preoperative physical, you find that he has a Mobitz II 2nd degree heart block, which has not been previously seen on prior ECGs. The patient has no other known medical problems and is on no medications.

Which of the following should be done regarding his heart condition prior to surgery?

A. Temporary pacemaker
B. Clinical EP study
C. Permanent pacemaker
D. Nothing else needs to be done, he may proceed to surgery

134.

A 35-year-old woman comes for a routine visit. She has no history of cardiac disease and is a nonsmoker. Her mother had a myocardial infarction at age 70.

On examination, blood pressure is normal, and body mass index is 28. LDL cholesterol is 169.

Diet and exercise are recommended.

On a follow-up visit in 3 months, she says she has tried to stick to her diet and is exercising twice a week. BMI and LDL cholesterol are unchanged.

Which of the following should you do next?

A. Add niacin
B. Add a statin
C. Check lipoprotein A
D. Add a beta-blocker
E. Refer for exercise and dietary counseling

135.

A 25-year-old pregnant woman at 25-weeks gestation presents for evaluation. The patient says that she thinks she had rheumatic fever as a child. She presents today in atrial fibrillation with pulmonary edema. You start therapy and order an echocardiogram.

Which of the following is the <u>most</u> likely etiology for her atrial fibrillation and pulmonary edema?

A. VSD
B. Coronary aneurysm
C. IHHS
D. Mitral stenosis
E. Atrial stenosis

136.

A 25-year-old man presents after having a syncopal episode while playing basketball this morning. He has no other symptoms and says that he feels fine now.

Physical Examination:

HEENT: Normal
Neck: Carotid pulse has a rapid upstroke and is bifid
Heart: RRR with a harsh, non-radiating midsystolic aortic murmur
Lungs: Clear to auscultation
Abdomen: Benign
GU: Normal male genitalia
Skin: No rash

On further testing you do some maneuvers. For example, when you have him perform a Valsalva maneuver, his murmur increases in intensity.

Which of the following statements is true?

    A. Coronary artery disease is likely.
    B. Several drugs have been shown to prolong survival in these patients.
    C. Beta-blockers and verapamil will not improve symptoms.
    D. The carotid pulse finding in this disorder is also seen in aortic stenosis.
    E. This patient has the most common cause of sudden death in exercising young people.

137.

A 50-year-old man 2 days ago had an acute MI. He is doing well and is recovering well after stent placement and angioplasty of his LAD coronary artery.

Past Medical History:
Peptic ulcer disease 5 years ago; on no medications
Diabetes mellitus for 20 years; on insulin
Gout 2 years ago; on no medications currently
Morbid obesity

Only other medicine he is on is an antihistamine for allergies.

Vital signs:
BP 130/70, P 90, RR 20, Temp 98° F
Besides his morbid obesity and early diabetic retinopathy, he has no abnormalities on physical examination.

Based on his history, which of the following is true?

    A. Aspirin is not recommended.
    B. An ACE inhibitor is contraindicated.
    C. The use of beta-blockers is acceptable even though he has diabetes.
    D. Short-acting calcium channel blockers have been shown to prolong survival post MI.
    E. Lipid lowering agents should be used only if his LDL is not below 150.

138.

A 50-year-old woman had an anterior wall MI 3 days ago. She has been doing well and has not had any problems since her admission. Suddenly she develops severe chest discomfort and collapses while walking in the hallway. Her BP is 70/palpable with thin thready pulses. She is hypoxic with an oxygen saturation of 88%. She now has a new loud holosystolic murmur along the left lower sternal border.

What has most likely happened?

- A. She has had a papillary muscle rupture.
- B. She has had a VSD occur.
- C. She has had another infarction.
- D. She has had a thrombus embolize to her brain.
- E. She has coronary artery rupture.

139.

A 50-year-old woman with shortness of breath and mental status changes is found at home. Multiple medications are in her home.

This is her initial ECG:

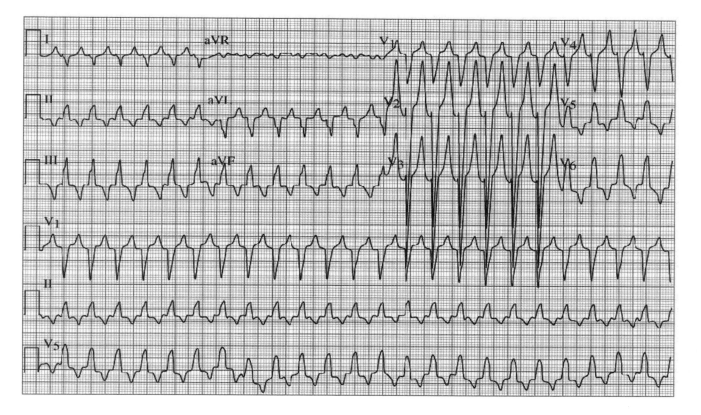

This ECG is done 30 minutes later after arrival to the ED. She is unconscious.

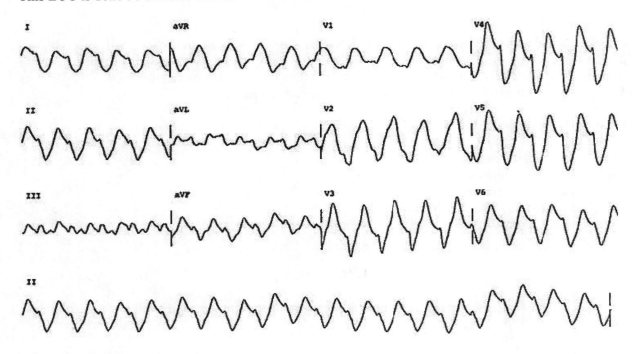

What is causing these abnormalities on ECG?

    A. She has asthma.
    B. She has constrictive pericarditis.
    C. She has severe aortic stenosis.
    D. She has hyperkalemia.
    E. She has hypothyroidism.

140.

Look at the ECG below and answer the question that follows.

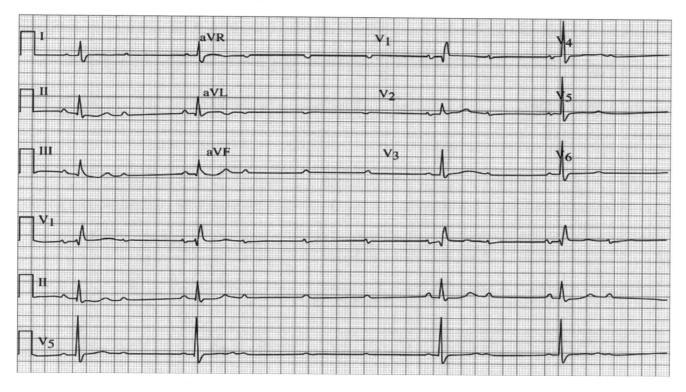

What type of arrhythmia is the ECG showing?

A. 1st degree AV block
B. 2nd degree AV block, Type 1
C. 2nd degree AV block, Type 2
D. Sinus arrhythmia
E. Sinus bradycardia

141.

A 45-year-old man presents with a large anterior myocardial infarction. He is hypotensive and tachycardic. Vital signs are seriously affected with a BP of 85/50 and a heart rate of 120. He begins to become unresponsive and appears to be deteriorating on arrival to the Emergency Department.

Which of the following treatments is inappropriate at this time?

A. Starting nitroprusside or nitroglycerin IV for afterload reduction
B. Placement of an intraaortic balloon pump
C. Getting the patient to the cardiac cath lab immediately
D. Placement of a Swan-Ganz catheter to monitor pressures and output
E. Starting inotropic agents (dopamine or dobutamine)

142.

You are seeing a 22-year-old for the first time for a pre-work physical exam. The patient reports he has had a few ear infections but is otherwise very healthy. His immunizations are up-to-date. On physical examination his vital signs are normal. Everything appears fine except you hear a systolic ejection murmur best heard at the left upper sternal border.

Which of the following would make you suspect an atrial septal defect?

    A. Fixed split second sound
    B. Early systolic ejection click
    C. Cyanosis
    D. Midsystolic click
    E. Greater arterial pulses in the upper extremities compared to the lower

143.

What are the 4 components of tetralogy of Fallot?

    A. Large VSD, right ventricular outflow tract obstruction, overriding aorta, RVH
    B. Large VSD, left ventricular outflow tract obstruction, overriding aorta, LVH
    C. Large VSD, right ventricular outflow tract obstruction, overriding aorta, LVH
    D. ASD, VSD, patent ductus arteriosus, LVH
    E. ASD, right ventricular outflow tract obstruction, overriding aorta, RVH

144.

A 35-year-old presents to your office complaining of palpitations. These occur most often when she drinks coffee. She has never had syncope. The palpitations can last up to 3–5 minutes and spontaneously resolve.

Past Medical History: Negative

Social History:
Married with 1 child
Smokes 2 packs/day of cigarettes

Family History:
Mother 60 with HTN
Father 50 with HTN

Review of Systems: Negative

Physical Examination:
Vitals: BP 130/70, P 90, RR 16, Temp 98.8° F, Ht. 5'1", Wt 230 lbs

HEENT:
PERRLA, EOMI
TMs: Clear
Throat: Clear

Neck: Supple
Heart: RRR without murmurs, rubs, or gallops
Lungs: CTA
Abdomen: Benign
Extremities: No cyanosis, clubbing, or edema

Resting ECG in your office is normal.

Which of the following would be the most useful test in evaluation of this patient?

A. Stress test
B. Left heart catheterization
C. Holter study
D. Right heart catheterization
E. Echocardiogram

145.

A 22-year-old college student seeks a pre-employment physical from you prior to applying for the position of ski instructor at the Crisp Ski Resort in Vail, CO. You note his tall thin habitus and obtain height and arm-span measurements of 73" each. Your examination documents a Grade II/VI systolic ejection "flow" murmur in the pulmonary outflow tract. Additionally he has fixed splitting of the second heart sound. His EKG demonstrates right axis deviation, and there are prominent R-waves in Lead V1 with an R:S ratio of [1.4:1].

His apparent right ventricular hypertrophy (RVH) is probably a result of which of the following?

A. Cystic fibrosis
B. Primary pulmonary hypertension
C. Ostium secundum atrial septal defect (ASD)
D. Membranous ventricular septal defect (VSD)
E. Type A Wolff-Parkinson-White syndrome (WPW)

146.

The history and electrocardiographic findings of various patients are listed below.

Which of the following patients is likely to benefit the most from thrombolytic therapy?

A. A 40-year-old man with the onset of chest pain four hours ago who has small Q waves and 3 mm of ST segment depression in leads II, III, and aVF
B. A 60-year-old woman with a recent onset of mild right hemiparesis and 2 hours of chest pain with an ECG showing no Q waves and 4 mm of ST segment elevation from leads V1 to V6, and 2 mm of ST elevation in leads I and aVF
C. A 60-year-old man with two previous coronary bypass surgeries and 2 hours of chest pain who has 4 mm of ST segment depression and new T wave inversion in leads V1 to V4
D. A 68-year-old woman with the onset of chest pain 2 hours ago with tall R waves and ST segment depression in leads V1 and V2
E. A 50-year-old man with the onset of chest pain 2 hours ago and a new left bundle branch block

147.

A 60-year-old man presents to the Emergency Department with symptoms of increasingly frequent chest pains. He says that the pain used to occur only with significant physical activity, but the last 3 nights he has been waking up with chest pain. He says that he gets lightheaded with the chest pain on exertion and needs to sit down for the pain to go away. The pain at night will usually subside after 5 or 10 minutes, but last night the pain lasted 20 minutes. He previously smoked 3 packs-a-day of cigarettes but said he quit last week. Cardiac enzymes are negative, but ECG shows ST segment elevation in anterior chest leads. In the ED, he has recurrence of his chest pain.

Based on this history, what is the next step in the workup?

    A. Thallium exercise stress test.
    B. Cardiac catheterization.
    C. Echocardiogram.
    D. Treadmill stress test; images are not required with his history.
    E. Ask him about depression as an etiology of his symptoms.

148.

A 35-year-old woman is 16 weeks pregnant. Her BP is 170/110, and her urinalysis shows she has 2+ proteinuria. Otherwise she has no complaints and is referred by her obstetrician for treatment of her hypertension.

Of the following, which is the best agent to use?

    A. Lisinopril
    B. Hydrochlorothiazide
    C. Nitroprusside drip
    D. Methyldopa
    E. Fosinopril

149.

A 55-year-old man received tissue plasminogen activator for an ST segment elevation myocardial infarction (STEMI). Three days later he had an episode of similar chest pain, relieved in 10 minutes by sublingual nitroglycerin.

Physical examination demonstrates a pericardial friction rub.

An ECG shows nonspecific ST-T wave changes.

Which of the following procedures should be done next?

    A. Coronary angiography
    B. Treatment with nonsteroidal antiinflammatory drugs
    C. Treatment with prednisone
    D. An exercise stress test with nuclear perfusion imaging
    E. An adenosine stress test with nuclear perfusion imaging

150.

Here is a short knowledge question that they will occasionally still throw at you on the Boards. If you don't know, guess. And to help your thinking—think of all the patients you have had on digoxin therapy. Which of these things have you never seen with digitalis? Or another way to think about it—you know of drugs that cause some of these side effects and are classically described. Is digitalis one that even comes up on your radar screen for this finding?

All of the following can be a side effect of digitalis toxicity <u>except</u>:

A. Headaches
B. Blurred vision
C. Gingival hyperplasia
D. Nausea and vomiting
E. Arrhythmias

151.

Here are normal pressures: RA Pressure: 0–5; Pulmonary Artery Pressure: 12–28/3–13; Pulmonary Capillary Wedge Pressure: 3–11.

Which of the following values would be associated with constrictive pericarditis?

	RA Pressure	Pulmonary Artery Pressure	Pulmonary Capillary Wedge Pressure
A.	16	75/30	11
B.	16	35/15	16
C.	16	99/29	28
D.	16	45/22	20
E.	16	22/12	10

152.

An 80-year-old man has had recent syncope that appears to be exercise-induced. He is now hospitalized for congestive heart failure. He has developed progressive shortness of breath for the past four days and increasing pedal edema. He tried increasing his usual dose of furosemide, without relief.

Past Medical History:	No prior hospitalizations for CHF
	History of coronary artery disease; coronary bypass grafting 5 years ago
	Hypertension for 30 years; currently on fosinopril 20 mg q day and furosemide 20 mg q day
	NIDDM; diet controlled

Social History:	Widowed 4 years ago
	Lives alone in a trailer
	Drinks 2 six-packs/beer a week for 30 years
	Smokes 1/2 pack a day of cigarettes; occasional cigar
	Veteran of WWII

Family History:	Mother and Father died at early ages of unknown causes
	Brother died at age 68 of MI
	Brother died at age 68 of MI
	Sister died at age 68 of MI
	3 sons; all with hypertension

Review of Systems: Deferred for this question (whew, aren't you glad? So is the question writer!)
Physical Examination: Well-developed, well-nourished man in mild distress
BP 163/80 mmHg, P 80, RR 18, Temp 98.4° F

HEENT: PERRLA, EOMI, bilateral cataracts (mild)
TMs: Clear
Throat: Clear
Neck: Supple, +JVD to 8 cm
Heart: RRR with III/VI harsh systolic murmur
Lungs: Bilateral crackles to mid lung fields
Abdomen: Bowel sounds present; no fluid wave; liver down about 5 cm below right costal margin
Extremities: No cyanosis; mild clubbing present; 3+ pitting edema to knee
GU: Mild scrotal edema

Laboratory: Echocardiogram: Disproportionately thickened ventricular septum and systolic anterior motion of the mitral valve

Based on your findings, which of the following is likely to be present?

A. Radiation of the murmur to the carotids
B. Delayed carotid upstroke
C. Signs of mitral stenosis
D. Decrease of the murmur with handgrip
E. Reduced left ventricular ejection fraction

153.

A 45-year-old woman comes in for her routine checkup. She has not had any problems and relates that she is doing well. She is not aware of any problems except she says that her ankles swell frequently, and that this has just started to occur.

| Past Medical History: | Essentially negative |
| | Delivered 6 children by normal spontaneous vaginal delivery |

| Meds: | None |

Social History:	Lives with her husband and 6 children in Lyme, CT
	Drinks a 6-pack of beer/week
	Smokes 2 packs/cigarettes daily
	Works as a weather forecaster

Family History:	Mother with CHF diagnosed at age 50
	Father with CHF diagnosed at age 50
	Brother 51 y/o good health

Review of Systems: No shortness of breath
                      Chronic cough especially in the morning for years
                      No edema of the hands or elsewhere noted
                      No orthopnea
                      No dyspnea on exertion or at rest
                      No weight gain or weight loss

Physical Examination:
     Vitals: Ht 5'5", Wt 120, BP 110/80, Temp 98° F, RR 12, P 88

     HEENT: PERRLA, EOMI, Discs sharp
     TMs: Clear
     Throat: Clear
     Neck: Supple, no masses
        Jugular venous pulse is 3 cm H_2O
        Hepatojugular reflux is negative
     Heart: RRR without murmurs, rubs, or gallops
     Lungs: CTA
     Abdomen: Bowel sounds present; no ascites; no masses
     Extremities: 2+ pitting edema to just past the ankle area bilaterally
        No cyanosis, clubbing noted

All of the following should be considered in the differential <u>except</u>:

  A. Pelvic thrombophlebitis
  B. Right heart failure
  C. Venous varicosities
  D. Cyclic edema
  E. Hypoalbuminemia

154.

A 41-year-old man without significant medical history presents for his annual physical. He has an ECG as a routine test required by his employer—the U.S. Postal Service. The ECG shows 2 premature ventricular complexes (PVCs) within the 12-lead tracing.

Which of the following is <u>not</u> true?

  A. PVCs such as these can cause symptoms.
  B. Both the frequency and the nature of PVCs can correlate with increased mortality in patients with known coronary artery disease.
  C. The frequency of PVCs increases with age.
  D. This patient's PVCs predict a higher incidence of cardiac mortality.
  E. 60% of men have PVCs on 24-hour Holter monitoring.

155.

T.L., a 17-year-old female, presents to clinic for her routine sports physical. She is finishing her junior year in high school and has been receiving offers from several colleges for soccer. This is your first time to see her. She has been doing well with no real concerns, but the mother does mention that T.L. gets dizzy and lightheaded sometimes when playing soccer. It usually occurs after playing for 30 minutes or longer. She does not have chest pain with exercise but sometimes feels nauseated. She has never passed out. There is no family history of sudden death.

PMH: Significant for migraines at age 6 but no longer has problems with that
Immunizations: UTD
Social: Lives in the city with her parents and 2 siblings. No pets. No smoking.

Physical Exam:
Vitals: Weight 136 pounds (70th percentile), height 63.5 inches (45th percentile)
BP 104/62   Pulse 52
      HEENT: Within normal limits
      Heart: Regular rate and rhythm, no murmur, normal pulses in all limbs
      Lungs: CTA in all lung fields, no wheezing
      Abdomen: Non-tender, no masses, no HSM
      Extremities: Strong pulses, no edema
      GU: Normal female, Tanner 5
      Skin: Warm, dry, no rash
      Lab: Hemoglobin 15.6

What would your next course of action be?

    A. ECG
    B. Reassurance to mother that the patient is just fine
    C. Have the patient take iron supplements and recheck in 2 months
    D. EEG
    E. Tell the patient she is not drinking enough and have her drink Gatorade 30 minutes prior to and during the game

156.

Jen, a 15-year-old female, presents to your office for a routine visit. She is starting high school this year, and there are no concerns. She has never been hospitalized. She is due for her booster tetanus immunization; otherwise her immunizations are up-to-date. Review of systems is negative.

Physical Exam: Weight and height are both between the 10th and 25th percentile
HEENT is within normal limits
Heart with II/VI systolic murmur heard best at left sternal border
Radial pulses 2+, femoral pulses 1+, BP 100/65
Lungs are clear
Abdomen is benign

What would be your immediate next step?

A. Measure blood pressure in all four limbs
B. Heart catheterization
C. Begin prostaglandin E1
D. Barium swallow
E. ECG

157.

Which of the following cardiac conditions requires dental prophylaxis?

A. Prosthetic mitral valve.
B. Hypertrophic cardiomyopathy (HCM).
C. Mitral valve prolapse with regurgitation seen on echocardiogram.
D. Bicuspid aortic valve.
E. All of the choices require dental prophylaxis.

158.

26-year-old Caucasian female is referred by her gynecologist because of hypertension. The gynecologist noticed that her blood pressure was in the 160–170/95–105 range on several readings three months ago, so her birth control pills were discontinued. Her BP has remained elevated. Her medical history is otherwise negative, and she has no FH of hypertension. PE: BP 164/104 in both arms, funduscopic exam is normal, there is no S_4 or bruits. Labs: Na 140, K 3.8, Cl 104, CO_2 26, BUN 11, Cr 0.7. EKG, biochemistry profile, U/A are normal.

A renal angiogram shows the following:

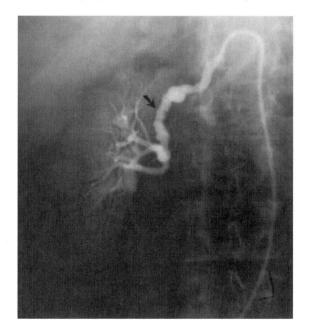

Which of the following agents would be the most appropriate initial therapy?

    A. Spironolactone
    B. Thiazide diuretic
    C. Amiloride
    D. Angiotensin converting enzyme inhibitor
    E. Beta-blocker

159.

A 28-year-old Internal Medicine resident presents with complaint of chest pain. He describes the pain as sharp, stabbing, intermittent, and radiating to his left chest. On occasion he also has some dysphagia.

Social History: Currently on Cardiology rotation; under lots of stress
                Recently separated from his wife
                Mother died last month

Family History: Mother with MI last month at age of 70
                Father with MI 2 years ago at age 68
                Brother healthy
                Sister healthy

Physical Examination:
    HEENT: Normal
    Neck: Supple, no masses
    Heart: RRR with I/VI flow murmur
    Lungs: Clear to auscultation
    Abdomen: + BS, benign
    Extremities: No rashes

He went to his fellow residents on various rotations and got the following tests done:
Stress test: Normal
EGD: Normal
Esophageal motility: Mostly normal peristalsis, but with 37% simultaneous contractions

On further questioning he tells you:
His dysphagia is for solids and liquids but especially cold liquids.

Based on his personal history, family history, physical findings, and laboratory studies, which of the following is true?

    A. Atypical angina is a likely diagnosis.
    B. Botox therapy is recommended.
    C. If a barium swallow is done, it usually is normal but can show a "corkscrew" pattern for this diagnosis.
    D. He has Plummer-Vinson syndrome.
    E. He should have a workup for scleroderma.

160.

A 74-year-old lethargic man is brought to the ED complaining of nausea, vomiting, and abdominal pain. He has been having vague muscle and joint pains for several days prior to admission. On exam, he has hyperreflexia, and you notice that he has fasciculations of the tongue. An electrocardiogram shows a shortened QT interval.

What is the most likely cause of his lethargy?

    A. Hypercalcemia
    B. Hypocalcemia
    C. Hyperkalemia
    D. Hypokalemia
    E. Carbon monoxide poisoning

161.

Determine the axis of the following ECG.

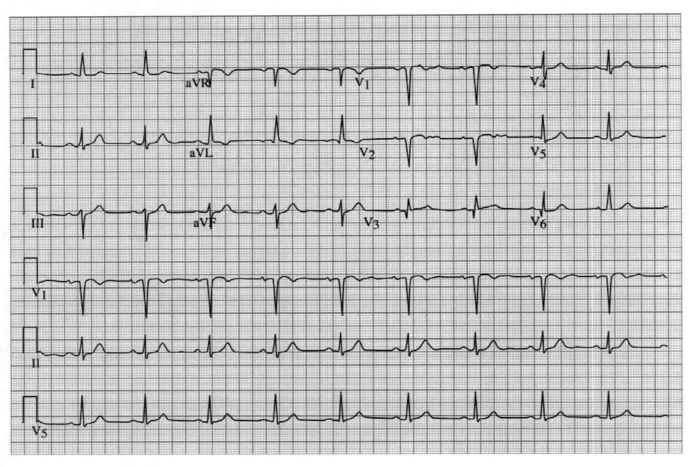

- A. Left axis deviation
- B. Right axis deviation
- C. Normal axis
- D. Can't tell
- E. Extreme right axis deviation

162.

Determine the axis for the following ECG.

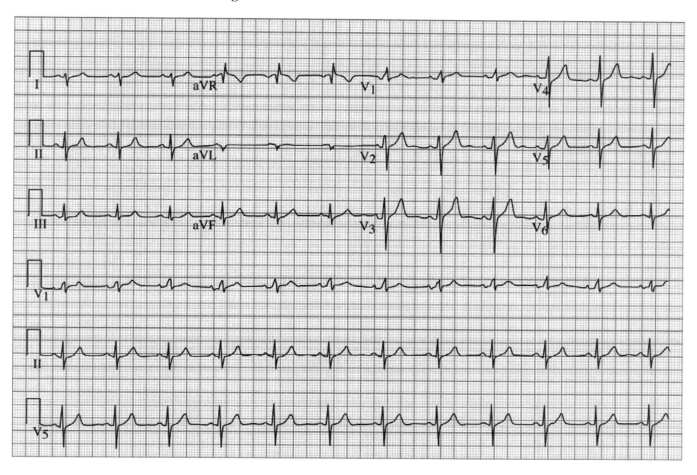

A. Left axis
B. Right axis
C. Normal axis
D. Can't tell
E. Isoelectric

163.

What is the finding in the following ECG?

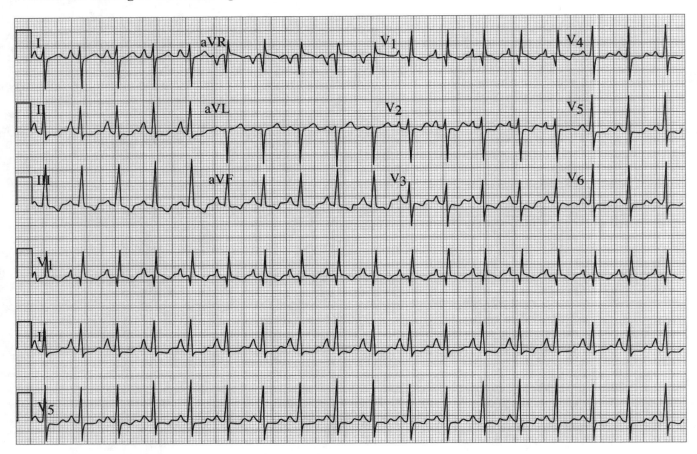

A. Right atrial enlargement
B. Left atrial enlargement
C. Right bundle branch block
D. Atrial fibrillation
E. Ventricular fibrillation

164.

What is the finding in this ECG?

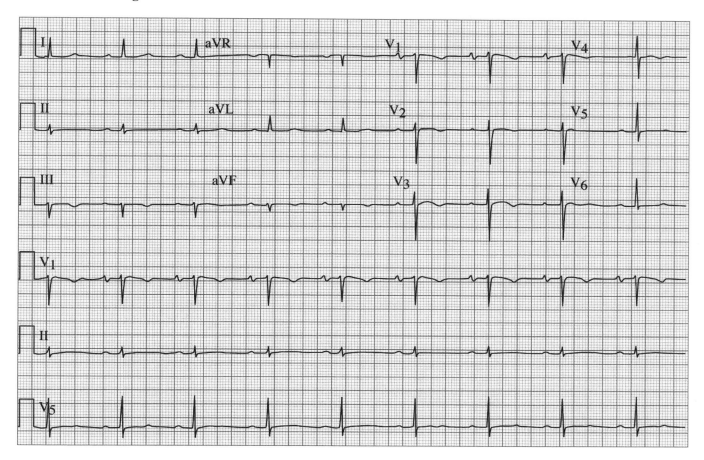

A. Left atrial enlargement
B. Right atrial enlargement
C. Atrial fibrillation
D. Ventricular fibrillation
E. Right bundle branch block

165.

What is the abnormality on this ECG?

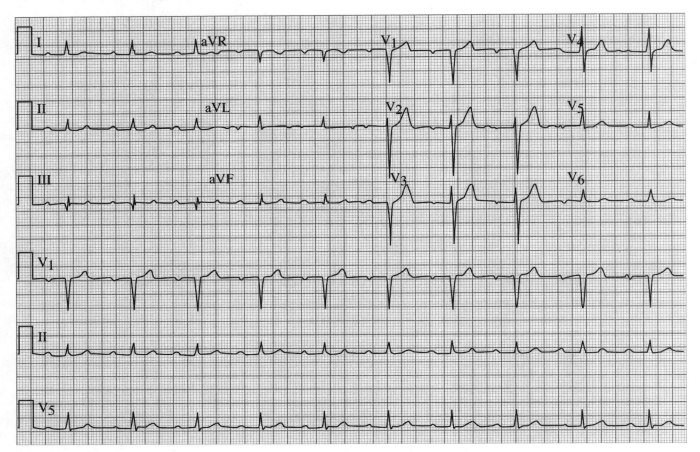

A. 1st degree heart block
B. 2nd degree heart block, Type 1
C. 2nd degree heart block, Type 2
D. 3rd degree heart block
E. Atrial fibrillation

166.

What is the abnormality on this ECG?

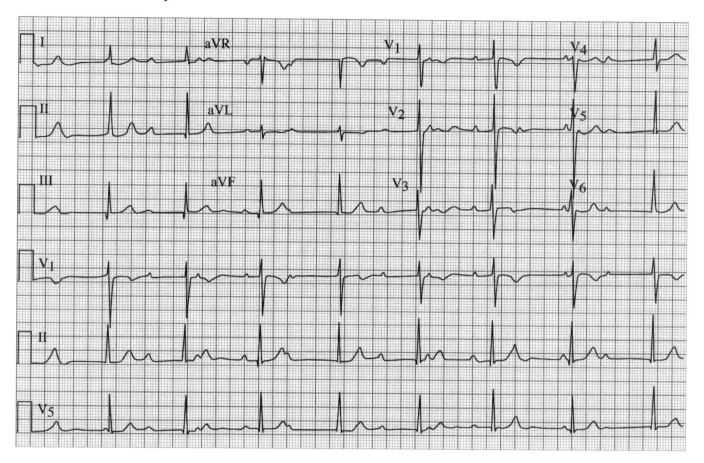

A. 1st degree heart block
B. 2nd degree heart block, Type 1
C. 2nd degree heart block, Type 2
D. 3rd degree heart block
E. Atrial fibrillation

167.

What is the abnormality on this ECG?

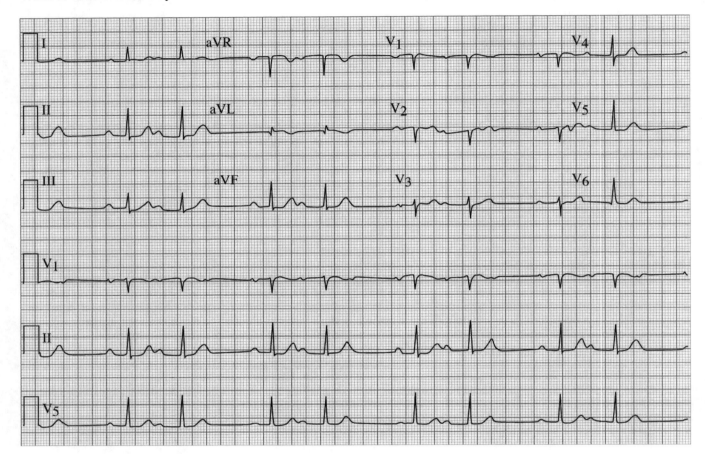

A. 1st degree heart block
B. 2nd degree heart block, Type 1
C. 2nd degree heart block, Type 2
D. 3rd degree heart block
E. Atrial fibrillation

168.

What is the abnormality in this ECG?

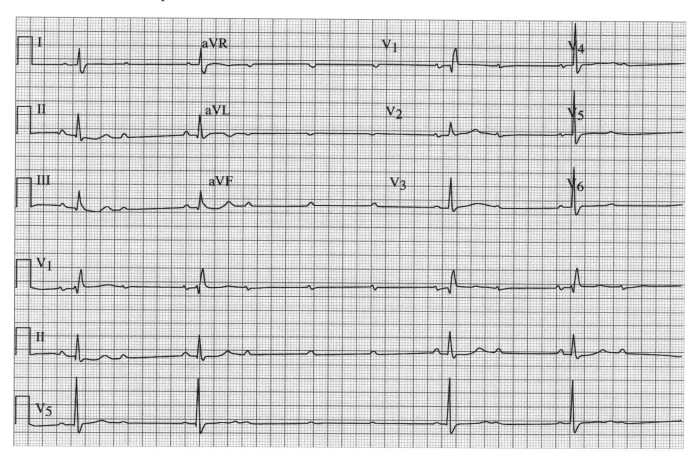

A. 1st degree heart block
B. 2nd degree heart block, Type 1
C. 2nd degree heart block, Type 2
D. 3rd degree heart block
E. Atrial fibrillation

169.

How do you interpret the following ECG?

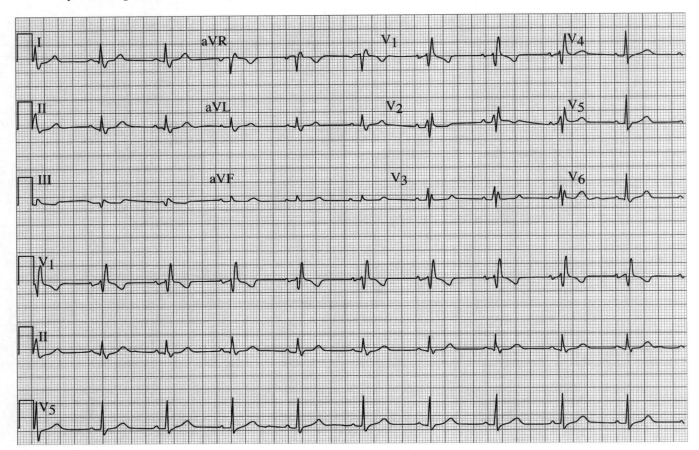

A. 1st degree AV block
B. Atrial fibrillation
C. Left bundle branch block
D. Right bundle branch block
E. 2nd degree AV block, Type 1

170.

How do you interpret this ECG?

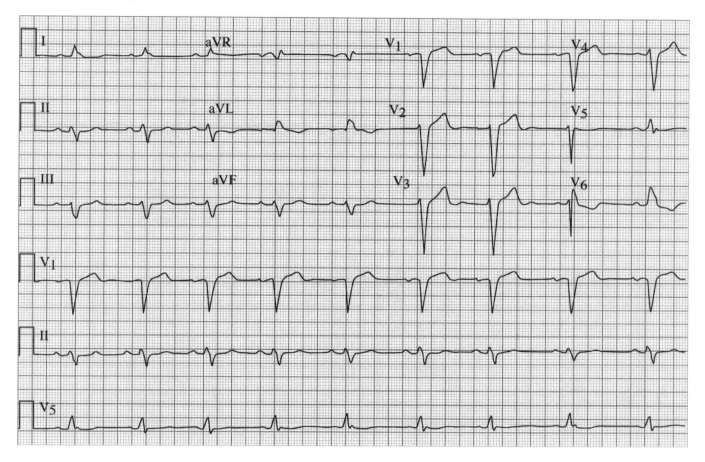

A. 1st degree AV block
B. Atrial fibrillation
C. Left bundle branch block
D. Right bundle branch block
E. 2nd degree AV block, Type 1

171.

How do you interpret this ECG?

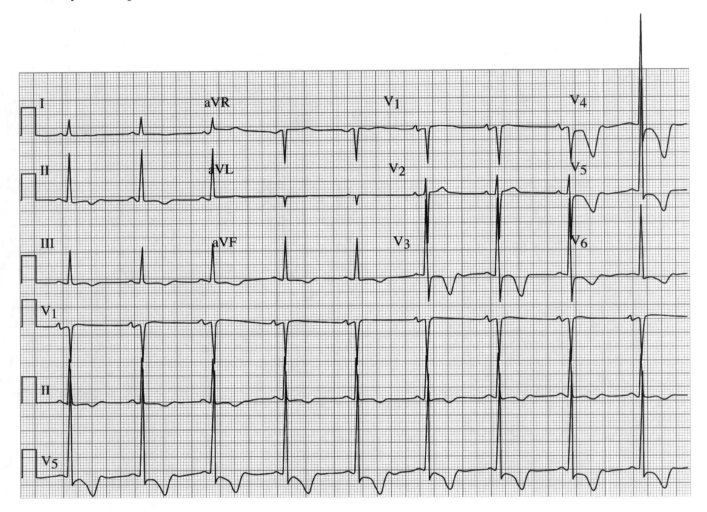

- A. Left bundle branch block
- B. Right bundle branch block
- C. Left ventricular hypertrophy
- D. Right ventricular hypertrophy
- E. 2nd degree AV block, Type 1

172.

How do you interpret this ECG?

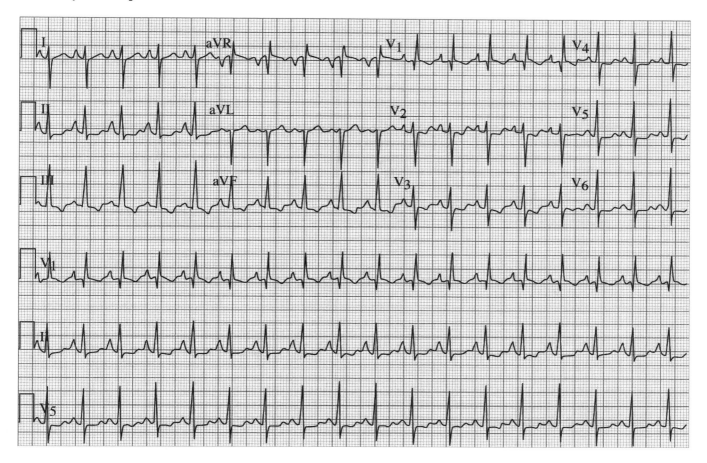

A. Left bundle branch block
B. Left axis deviation
C. Left ventricular hypertrophy
D. Right ventricular hypertrophy
E. 2nd degree AV block, Type 1

173.

A patient presents with acute onset of shortness of breath.

What does the following ECG suggest as a possible etiology for the shortness of breath?

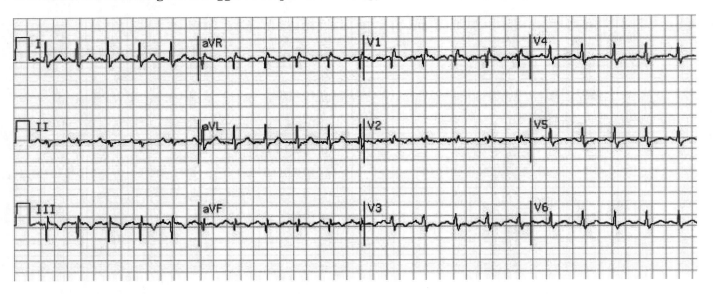

   A. Tamponade
   B. Constrictive pericarditis
   C. Pulmonary embolism
   D. Mitral valve prolapse
   E. Trauma to the chest

174.

What is the location of this recent MI?

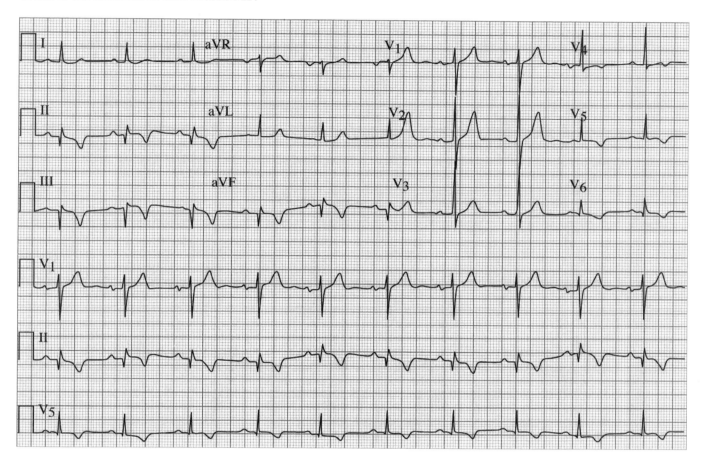

- A. Anterior MI
- B. Anterior-septal MI
- C. Inferior MI
- D. No MI
- E. Posterior MI

175.

Where is the location of this MI?

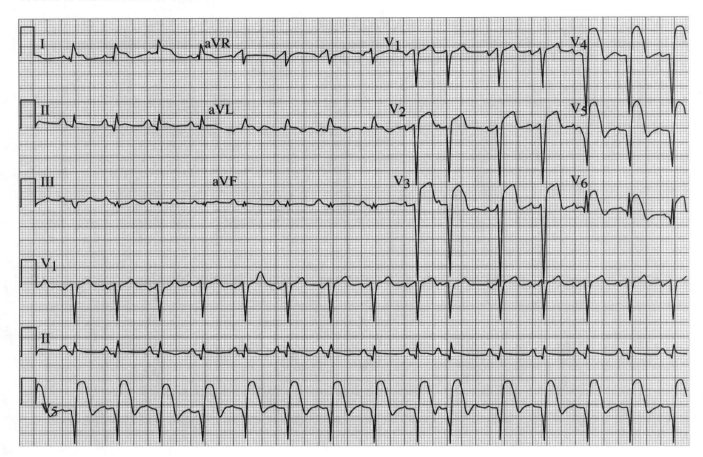

A. Anterior-lateral MI
B. Inferior MI
C. No MI
D. Posterior MI
E. Tiny septal MI

176.

What is your interpretation of this ECG?

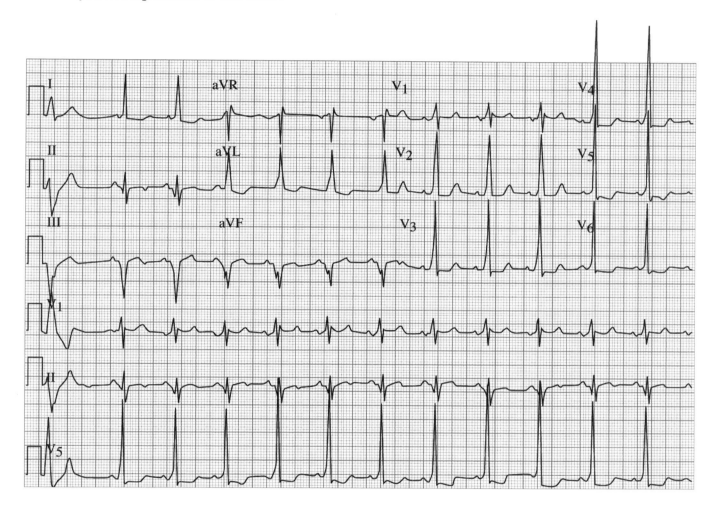

A. 1ˢᵗ degree AV block
B. 2ⁿᵈ degree AV block, Type 2
C. Acute anterior MI
D. Wolff-Parkinson-White
E. Normal

177.

Which of the following is <u>not</u> associated with ST-segment depression?

A. Myocardial ischemia
B. Digitalis toxicity
C. ST depression in V1 with a posterior MI
D. Hypokalemia
E. Cocaine abuse

178.

On the Board exam, look for patients with acute tricyclic overdose.

What QT interval abnormality do you expect in these individuals?

    A. Prolonged QT.
    B. Short QT.
    C. No change in the QT.
    D. Can be either prolonged or short QT.
    E. QT cannot be determined in these individuals.

179.

A 64-year-old male had an inferior STEMI and was treated with aspirin, beta-blockers, an angiotensin converting enzyme inhibitor, and a statin. He was standing at the nurse's station when telemetry showed the following:

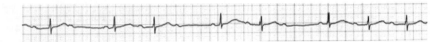

Which of the following should you do?

    A. Insert a temporary transvenous pacemaker
    B. Refer for permanent pacemaker implantation
    C. Refer for an electrophysiology study
    D. Decrease the beta-blocker dose
    E. Refer for coronary angiography

180.

A 74-year-old female comes to the Emergency Department with chest pain and dyspnea and is found to have a non-ST segment elevation MI (NSTEMI).

Physical exam and chest x-ray show pulmonary edema

She is given a beta-blocker, intravenous morphine, sublingual nitroglycerin, and 160 mg of intravenous furosemide.

She initially improves but one hour later becomes hypotensive. A right heart catheter is inserted and the following pressures are obtained:

Location	Pressure (mmHg)
Right Atrium	2
Pulmonary Artery	20/10
Pulmonary Capillary Wedge	6

Which of the following treatments is appropriate?

A. Insert an intraaortic balloon pump
B. Refer for emergency percutaneous coronary intervention
C. Fibrinolytic therapy
D. Normal saline infusion
E. Blood cultures and empiric antibiotics

181.

What is the arrhythmia depicted in this ECG?

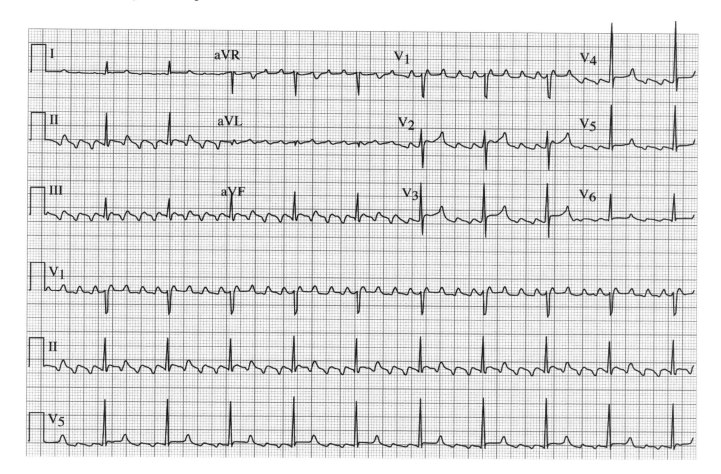

A. Atrial fibrillation
B. Atrial flutter
C. Ventricular tachycardia
D. Ventricular fibrillation
E. Wolff-Parkinson-White

182.

What arrhythmia does this ECG depict?

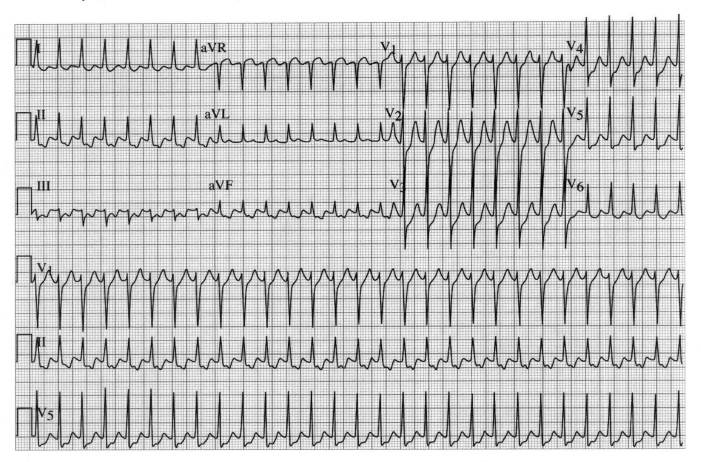

- A. Atrial flutter
- B. Atrial fibrillation
- C. Paroxysmal supraventricular tachycardia (PSVT)
- D. Ventricular fibrillation
- E. Ventricular tachycardia

183.

What is the arrhythmia depicted by this ECG?

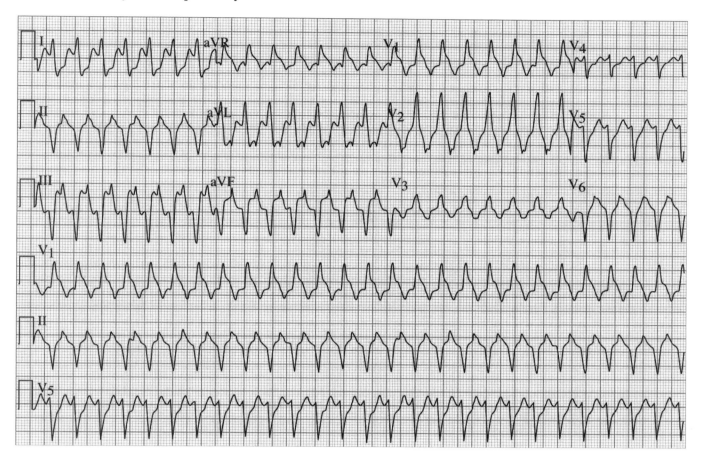

A. Atrial flutter
B. Atrial fibrillation
C. Paroxysmal supraventricular tachycardia (PSVT)
D. Ventricular fibrillation
E. Ventricular tachycardia

184.

What is the arrhythmia depicted by this ECG?

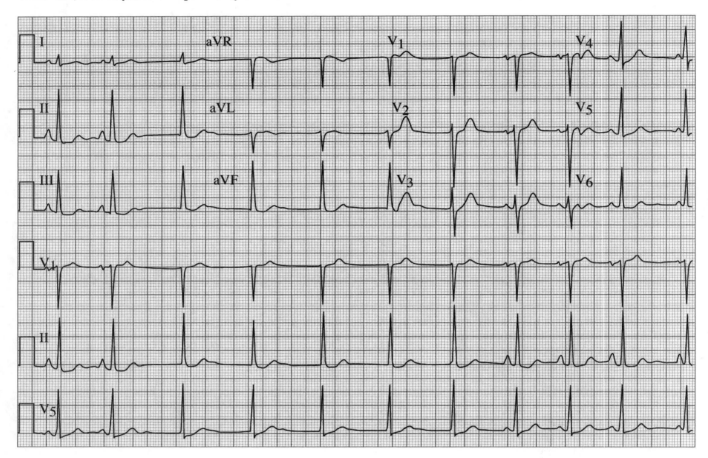

A. 1st degree AV block
B. 2nd degree AV block
C. 3rd degree AV block
D. Junctional rhythm
E. Wandering atrial pacemaker

185.

A 56-year-old male presents with a systolic murmur.

Echocardiography shows a left ventricular ejection fraction of 50%, an LV systolic dimension of 60 mm, severe mitral valve prolapse, and severe mitral regurgitation.

He exercises for 4 minutes on a Bruce protocol, to a peak heart rate of 105, and peak blood pressure of 130/80, stopping because of dyspnea. Rest and peak exercise ECGs follow.

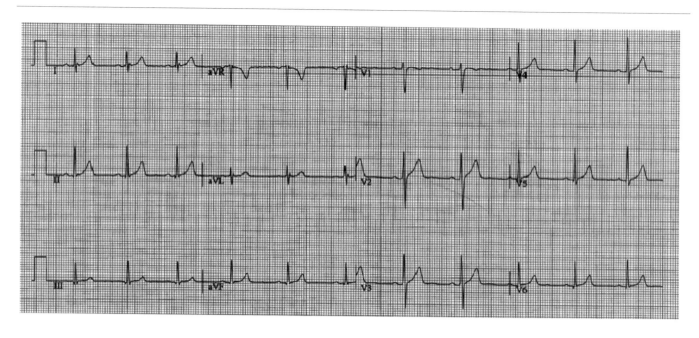

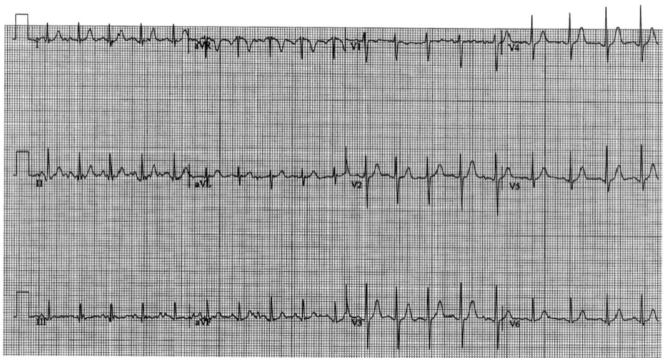

Which of the following should be done next?

A. Dobutamine stress echo
B. Observe for 6 more months and repeat the evaluation
C. Refer for mitral valve replacement
D. Therapy with beta-blockers

186.

A 43-year-old male complains of intermittent palpitations and increasing dyspnea. He is found to have a systolic murmur that becomes softer on passive leg raising and deep inspiration and louder during the strain phase of the Valsalva maneuver.

Which of the following is the correct diagnosis?

A. Aortic stenosis
B. Tricuspid regurgitation
C. Mitral regurgitation
D. Membranous VSD
E. Hypertrophic obstructive cardiomyopathy

INFECTIOUS DISEASE

187.

A 70-year-old woman presents with cellulitis of her left foot. She does not have diabetes. She thinks she scratched her toe while walking barefoot in her rock garden at home. Otherwise she is without complaint. You note that her skin is slightly red without oozing or abnormal characteristics. She is not allergic to any medications, but leather makes her itch. She is afebrile. She has no history of MRSA and has not been in a hospital setting.

Which of the following is the best antibiotic to treat the most likely organism?

    A. Ceftriaxone
    B. Ceftazidime
    C. Cefazolin
    D. Gentamicin
    E. Erythromycin

188.

Maria Fitz-Hugh-Curtis, a dancer by night, a part-time petting zoo employee by day, presents with a 2-day history of diarrhea. She reports some blood in the stool and has had a low-grade fever. She lives alone and says that coworkers at the petting zoo have also had diarrhea; no one at the dancing club has had diarrhea that she knows of. When asked about the animals at the petting zoo, she rattles off a long list including goats, pigs, caterpillars, iguanas, mice, gerbils, rabbits, ducks, chickens, swans, donkeys, llamas, camels, horses, cows, and snakes. WHEW! You then ask her which animals in particular does she have contact with. She reports that she likes to deal only with the iguanas, snakes, and goats.

Assuming that her diarrhea is infectious and due to bacteria, what organism is most likely, based on her animal exposure?

    A. *Shigella*
    B. *Klebsiella*
    C. *Francisella*
    D. *Neisseria*
    E. *Salmonella*

189.

A 19-year-old college student in Arkansas is studying animal husbandry. (For you non-farming folks this involves learning about animals whose purpose is mainly to provide meat for the table and includes beef cattle, sheep, and meat goats; this is in contrast to dairy animals. Anyway, back to the question at hand.) He presents with a swollen inguinal lymph node of 3 days duration with fever. He likes to hunt and has been in the rural woods of northern Arkansas every weekend for the past 3 months. He has removed numerous ticks from his body. At one tick bite location he has a new ulceration.

What is the likely organism responsible?

A. *Brucella*
B. *Klebsiella*
C. *Francisella*
D. *Legionella*
E. *Yersinia*

190.

A 38-year-old-man from rural Missouri presents with a four-day history of fever, mild sore throat, and fatigue. He enjoys hiking in the Ozark Mountains of southern Missouri and denies knowledge of tick bites but has seen a few ticks on his dog. He enjoys swimming with his dog in a local pond. He denies lymphadenopathy and other symptoms. He reports no rash.

Physical examination is unremarkable except for mild hepatosplenomegaly.
Laboratory is done and shows a WBC of 1,500 with 60% lymphs, 10% bands, and 20% neutrophils. He is anemic with a hemoglobin of 10 mg/dL, and his platelet count is 55,000.

Which of the following is the most appropriate study to diagnose the infection causing his illness?

A. Lymph node biopsy
B. Skin test
C. Blood culture
D. Acute and convalescent antibody titers
E. Urine culture

191.

A 40-year-old woman lives in a town of 150,000 people in Wisconsin. She reports a 3-day history of diarrhea that is non-bloody in character. This is the 10th person you have seen in the office today with similar history, and your nurse has received at least 10 additional phone calls about similar episodes. Your colleague says that she has seen a bunch of diarrhea cases in the past day. You call the local health department and they report that the diarrhea is citywide, and they are working on figuring out the etiology. They do report that routine stool cultures are negative so far. Stool ova and parasites are pending.

What test is most likely to be positive and give a clue as to the etiology?

A. *Salmonella* specific antigen
B. Acid-fast stain of the stool
C. *Chlamydia* cultures
D. Fungal stain of the stool
E. Urine antigen test

192.

A 60-year-old woman with poorly controlled diabetes mellitus presents with a 2-day history of nasal stuffiness and frequent nose bleeds. She has some sinus tenderness on examination, and when you look into her nasal cavity, you see a small black necrotic area on the nasal turbinate.

Which of the following organisms should you be most concerned about?

  A. *Streptococcus pneumoniae*
  B. *Haemophilus influenzae* non-typeable
  C. *Mycobacterium nasalitum*
  D. *Mucor* species
  E. *Sporothrix schenckii*

193.

A 20-year-old woman who underwent a splenectomy in 2000 after an MVA resulted in splenic rupture presents for evaluation. She received vaccination against pneumococcus and *H. influenzae*. She has been visiting the islands off Massachusetts and presents with high fever to 105° F, shaking chills, and rigors. She is quite pale. Laboratory returns and shows a severe hemolytic anemia. You suspect a parasite.

What is the best way to diagnosis her infection?

  A. Blood culture
  B. Thick and thin blood smears
  C. Urine culture
  D. Stool culture
  E. CT scan of the head to look for cysts

194.

A 29-year-old woman resides in Brownsville, Texas. She has been noted to have a liver abscess that is felt to likely be due to *Entamoeba histolytica*.

What is the best way to determine if this is the likely etiology?

  A. Serology testing
  B. Aspirate the liver abscess
  C. Stool culture
  D. Stool ova and parasite examination
  E. String test

195.

A 40-year-old woman presents with genital lesions. They are itchy and painful and she has never had them before. In the past few months she has been dating a new boyfriend. They have had sexual intercourse on numerous occasions, and she reports the use of a diaphragm for birth control. Her menses have been normal, and she has not had any difficulties until this episode, which began yesterday.

On examination you confirm the diagnosis of herpes simplex (HSV) and begin her on a course of valacyclovir. She is concerned about her diagnosis of genital herpes and has several questions for you.

Which of the following is true regarding genital herpes infection?

A. If she were pregnant with active lesions, C-section would not be helpful.
B. It is possible for her to spread the virus to others even if lesions are not present.
C. Use of anti-HSV drugs will not be beneficial in preventing future outbreaks.
D. A Tzanck smear would be negative at this point.
E. HSV is an RNA virus.

196.

A 60-year-old RN has newly diagnosed herpes zoster infection. His infection is located on his right scapula and spreads laterally over 3–4 dermatomal areas. He is not immunocompromised and is otherwise healthy. He works in an outpatient clinic.

What can you tell him about his zoster infection?

A. A Tzanck smear would be negative.
B. This infection is due to reactivation of herpes simplex virus.
C. The duration of post-herpetic neuralgia may be decreased by using valacyclovir.
D. If he had presented last week, with a "zoster-prodrome" (e.g., pain before the rash appeared) you should have started him on anti-virals.
E. He may not return to work until all his lesions are crusted over.

197.

An 18-year-old freshman at Bowling Blue University in northeastern Lyme, Connecticut presents to you at the school infirmary with a 2-day history of fever, cough, runny nose, and conjunctivitis. He initially thought he had a cold since a friend of his had a similar illness 2 weeks ago. Last night, however, he developed a rash that began at the back of his neck and has started to spread downward. He denies tick bites and reports that he is not nor has he ever been sexually active.

On physical examination you note that his rash is maculopapular in appearance and indeed starts at his hairline and continues to his back and trunk. On examination of his oral mucosa, you note whitish spots on a red base.

Which of the following is true?

A. Immunize all immunocompetent people at the college born in or after 1957 with a live virus vaccine if you cannot document 2 vaccinations against this virus have been given previously.
B. Immunize everyone regardless of age or immunization history with a killed virus vaccine.
C. Notify unimmunized pregnant women exposed to this illness that they are at high risk for congenital malformations in their infants.
D. People with egg allergy should not receive the live virus vaccine.
E. Asymptomatic HIV-infected students at the college should not receive the vaccine.

198.

A 35-year-old woman presents for evaluation. She has a 5-year-old son with an infection diagnosed 2 weeks ago; he presented then with "slapped cheeks" and rash on his extremities. Today she complains of a mild rash and arthritis of her hands. The arthritis mainly involves the wrist and the proximal interphalangeal joints. She reports a good amount of pain associated with this arthritis.

Which of the following is true about her infection?

A. The arthritis is due to a bacterial superantigen.
B. Her arthritis will likely become superinfected with *Streptococcus pyogenes*.
C. The child is likely still contagious to other family members.
D. If she has sickle cell disease, she could be at risk for aplastic crisis.
E. Immunization could have prevented this from occurring.

199.

A 25-year-old woman is newly diagnosed with HIV. Her CD4+ count returns and is 165. Her HIV viral load is 100,000 copies/mL. However, she is asymptomatic.

Which of the following treatments do you recommend at this point?

A. Return in 6 months and if CD4 is below 150, start anti-retroviral therapy.
B. Offer her ZDV/D4T and efavirenz with TMP/SMX.
C. Offer her ZDV/D4T/ddC with TMP/SMX.
D. Offer her ZDV only since she might get pregnant in the next few months.
E. Offer her tenofovir, emtricitabine, and efavirenz with TMP/SMX.

200.

A 50-year-old IV drug abuser presents with new-onset murmur and fever. Blood cultures grow *Staphylococcus aureus* in 4 bottles.

What is the most common cause of cardiac death in people with her diagnosis?

A. Thromboembolism to the brain
B. Arrhythmia
C. Congestive heart failure
D. Valve failure
E. Papillary muscle dysfunction

201.

A 30-year-old woman with negative past medical history works in a daycare and provides care for 20 children a day. Most of the children are aged 1–3 years. Her husband brings her to the emergency room with fever and severe headache. She notes her neck is stiff and that while driving over to the hospital the sunlight "hurt her eyes." She has no known sick contacts except for the numerous runny noses and colds that the daycare children have on a daily basis.

Physical examination is significant for meningismus and a positive Kernig sign. She has marked photophobia. Her optic discs are well demarcated, and no signs of intracranial pressure are noted. She has no focal neurologic signs.

Which of the following treatments do you recommend?

    A. A CT scan should be performed before lumbar puncture is attempted.
    B. Attempt a quick lumbar puncture followed by immediate administration of IV vancomycin and IV ceftriaxone.
    C. Attempt a quick lumbar puncture followed by immediate administration of IV ceftriaxone.
    D. IV acyclovir should be administered immediately.
    E. If lumbar puncture cannot be done immediately, you should withhold IV antibiotics until you can get the CSF to ensure a proper culture.

202.

A 60-year-old alcoholic male visits the gulf coast of Texas on a frequent basis and enjoys eating raw oysters and drinking large quantities of beer. This year, he rented a fishing house on the beach and wades out daily to fish in the Gulf of Mexico.

He presents via ambulance with a 30-minute history of "feeling weak" and passing out. He is found by a friend in his home. He has skin lesions on his leg. His blood pressure is 76/20 with a pulse of 120. He is in presumed septic shock.

Which of the following is the likely organism causing his sepsis?

    A. *Clostridium difficile*
    B. *Pseudomonas aeruginosa*
    C. *Nocardia species*
    D. *Vibrio vulnificus*
    E. *Yersinia enterocolitica*

203.

A 60-year-old retiree, named Ken, is enjoying his first cruise in the Caribbean. The ship has been at sea for 2 days, and many passengers have complained of diarrhea, which the patient attributes to rough seas. He got a scopolamine patch from his doctor and has not felt the least bit nauseous. However, suddenly at 2 a.m. he awakens with the urge to defecate and has explosive diarrhea. This continues throughout the remaining night. He calls the ship's doctor but cannot get through because the line is busy. He manages to make it to the infirmary and notes 30–40 passengers in the hallway, all with similar symptoms.

What is the most likely etiology for this unfortunate diarrheal illness?

    A. Norovirus (formerly known as Norwalk virus)
    B. Rotavirus
    C. *Campylobacter jejuni*
    D. *Clostridium difficile*
    E. *Cyclospora*

204.

An 18-year-old high school student presents to the Emergency Department with a severe swollen left ankle. She notes that she had fever today and then had some "bumps" come up on her leg. The ankle became swollen this morning and has progressively gotten worse. She is sexually active but reports that her "boyfriend was a virgin like me" and denies any knowledge of STD exposure. She started her menses yesterday and it has been normal. She denies any trauma.

Physical examination is significant for a markedly swollen left ankle with frank arthritis and palpable edema. 2 small pustules are located above the ankle area.

What is the most likely etiology for her arthritis?

A. Parvovirus B19
B. HSV synovitis
C. *Streptococcus pyogenes*
D. *Staphylococcus aureus*
E. *Neisseria gonorrhoeae*

205.

A 28-year-old man with chicken pox presents in shock with a blood pressure of 70/50. He is noted to have a rash on his palms/soles and lower extremities. Laboratory returns and it appears that he has renal failure (creatinine 3.5 mg/dL); liver abnormalities (ALT 400, AST 450, PT 16); thrombocytopenia with platelets of 80,000; mucous membrane changes; and diarrhea. A blood culture grows an organism.

What is the likely etiology of his condition?

A. *Staphylococcus aureus*
B. *E. coli*
C. *Rickettsia rickettsii*
D. *Francisella tularensis*
E. *Streptococcus pyogenes*

206.

A 21-year-old college student presents with new onset of hearing loss. She reports that she has had gradual hearing loss for the past 2 weeks. About 6 months ago she noted a rash on her extremities with mild fever. The rash resolved and she has been well since. She works in a daycare. She has been sexually active with the same individual for the past 2 years and is monogamous. Neither she nor her boyfriend has had a sexually transmitted disease that she knows of. She lives in Georgia and has no knowledge of tick bites. She has 2 dogs.

Which of the following is the most likely explanation for her hearing loss?

A. Rubella
B. Rubeola
C. Lyme disease
D. *Treponema pallidum*
E. Leptospirosis

207.

A 36-year-old woman lives in Bogue Holler, Arkansas, on the Buffalo River. She works as a schoolteacher in the local elementary school that has an enrollment of 15. Last week while "gettin" the firewood for the classroom stove, she noticed that a tick was embedded in her right leg. She removed the tick and didn't think anything about it until 3 days later, when she noticed that she had a marked irritation and "swellin" in her groin. That evening she developed fever and severe malaise. She applied a poultice of sprouts, cayenne pepper, and Tabasco sauce, but it didn't get any better. She presents to you today for evaluation.

Physical exam reveals an ulcerated area at the tick bite with a 3x5 cm right inguinal lymph node. She has a temperature of 103.2° F. Besides that, she has poor dentition.

Which of the following is the most likely diagnosis?

  A. Lyme disease
  B. *Ehrlichia*
  C. Tularemia
  D. Plague
  E. *Bartonella henselae* infection

208.

Which of these antibiotics is effective for gram-negative killing even after the drug has fallen below the MIC?

  A. Erythromycin
  B. Vancomycin
  C. Nafcillin
  D. Gentamicin
  E. Azactam

209.

A 45-year-old woman with AML is undergoing chemotherapy. She is severely neutropenic and has now spiked a fever to 102° F. You start an initial "rule-out" sepsis workup and want to start antibiotics. You find no focus for her fever.

Which of the following antibiotics is the best choice for her?

  A. Ceftriaxone
  B. Ceftazidime
  C. Vancomycin and ceftriaxone
  D. Vancomycin and cefoxitin
  E. Vancomycin and clindamycin

210.

A 40-year-old man presents with stiff neck and fever of 1 hour duration. He is disoriented and is not able to answer questions. His partner states that he was well until this morning and that he was singing in the shower as he usually does. However, by lunch time when they were eating, he complained of the headache and he quickly deteriorated. He was not ill before this.

PMH: Negative

Social History: Works as a lounge singer in New York City

Family History: Non-contributory

Physical Examination:
BP 110/70, P 100, RR 30, Temp 103° F
Oriented only to person (thinks it is 1969 and Marsha Brady is his wife)

Exam is significant for:
Meningismus
Brudzinski and Kernig signs are present

It has been 20 minutes since he hit the ED door, and you have done all of this assessment rapidly. He has no focal neurologic findings on examination. His discs are sharp, and he has normal neurologic examination. Also you know that the rate of resistance to cephalosporins by a certain gram-positive diplococcus in your area is nearly 10%.

Based on this, which of the following do you recommend?

    A. Stat CT scan followed by LP, then IV ceftriaxone and IV clindamycin
    B. Immediate LP, followed by IV ceftriaxone and IV vancomycin
    C. Immediate LP, followed by IV vancomycin only for resistant organisms
    D. Stat CT scan followed by LP and IV ceftriaxone
    E. Immediate LP, followed by IV ceftriaxone

211.

Which of the following antibiotics should not be used in a pregnant woman?

    A. Azithromycin
    B. Vancomycin
    C. Oxacillin
    D. Ciprofloxacin
    E. Cefepime

212.

A 28-year-old man presents with high fever, aches, and pains and says he "feels like a Mack-truck ran over me this morning." You are aware of influenza B in the community and have seen multiple cases in the past week. He became acutely ill this morning about 4 hours ago.

Which of the following would be helpful in reducing his symptoms and diminishing his viral shedding?

A. Acyclovir.
B. Amantadine or rimantadine.
C. Rimantadine is effective, but amantadine is not as effective.
D. Oseltamivir.
E. Amantadine, rimantadine, or oseltamivir would be helpful.

213.

A 70-year-old man with chronic renal insufficiency presents for evaluation. He is on chronic hemodialysis, which he receives 3 days a week at his local dialysis center. Yesterday morning he developed a fever and comes in for his usual dialysis. He is not that ill but has a temperature of 101.5° F. His graft site looks fine and he is without other complaints. Physical examination is unremarkable. Blood cultures are taken and within 24 hours are growing an organism.

Which of the following organisms is most likely, given his current examination and findings?

A. Methicillin-sensitive *Staphylococcus epidermidis*.
B. Methicillin-resistant *Staphylococcus epidermidis*.
C. Methicillin-resistant *Streptococcus aureus*.
D. Methicillin-resistant *Streptococcus pneumoniae*.
E. A gram-negative organism is most likely.

214.

A 25-year-old woman presents in shock. She is noted to have fever, diarrhea, and is incoherent. On examination she has a flushed red appearance to her skin and her BP is 70/20. She is menstruating; her boyfriend denies knowledge of sexually transmitted disease. A few petechiae are noted on her extremities. Laboratory shows abnormal liver enzymes, hypocalcemia, and an elevated PT.

What is the most likely cause of her findings?

A. Urinary tract infection
B. Disseminated *Neisseria gonorrhoeae*
C. *E. coli* sepsis
D. Rocky Mountain spotted fever
E. Toxic shock syndrome

215.

A 3-week-old presents to the Emergency Department with signs of sepsis.

What is/are the appropriate antibiotic(s)?

- A. IV ceftriaxone alone is best.
- B. IV ampicillin and IV cefotaxime.
- C. IV ampicillin and IV chloramphenicol.
- D. IV ampicillin and IV clindamycin.
- E. IV ceftriaxone and oral ampicillin.

216.

A man from Arizona presents with an inguinal lymphadenopathy and fever. He is a hunter and lives in the desert.

Which of the following diseases is most likely in this man?

- A. Tularemia.
- B. *Ehrlichia.*
- C. Plague.
- D. *Pasteurella.*
- E. Either tularemia or plague is likely.

217.

A 35-year-old IV drug abuser presents with headache and fever. He is incoherent and you have difficulty getting a good history from him. He was in the ED 2 weeks ago for an alcohol binge; HIV testing at that time was negative. A CT scan is negative, and IV ceftriaxone and IV vancomycin are given in the ED before the CT scan. A lumbar puncture is performed and shows the following results:

CSF WBC 100 cells: 60% polys and 40% lymphs
CSF Protein: 170 mg/dL
CSF Glucose: 70 mg/dL with serum glucose of 100 mg/dL
CSF VDRL is negative
CSF cryptococcal antigen is negative

Based on these results, what can you say about his diagnosis?

- A. Bacterial meningitis has been excluded.
- B. Neurosyphilis is possible.
- C. Acute HIV is likely.
- D. Fungal meningitis is likely.
- E. Alcohol intoxication is likely responsible for the CSF findings.

218.

A 38-year-old man with AIDS (CD4 count is 20) presents for evaluation. He resides in Indiana and does not take any anti-HIV medications ("they make me sick"). He presents with fever and chills of several days duration. He notes that he has been weak and cannot walk up a flight of stairs without getting short of breath. Physical examination shows hepatosplenomegaly and a palatal ulcer. Laboratory is significant for pancytopenia with a WBC of 1,500, with hemoglobin of 7.0 mg/dL, and platelet count of 110,000.

Which of the following opportunistic infections is most likely the etiology?

A. Coccidioidomycosis
B. *Blastomyces* species
C. *Histoplasma capsulatum*
D. Tuberculosis
E. *Pneumocystis jiroveci (carinii)*

219.

A 65-year-old man with poorly controlled diabetes presents to the dentist for a routine examination, and while there his dentist notes a black growth in his nose (he is in the Trendelenburg position for his dental examination). The exam reveals a painless black ulcer in the nasal septum.

He immediately goes to his internist, who examines him and refers him immediately to the hospital for admission and ENT consult.

Which of the following is the likely diagnosis?

A. *Aspergillus* infection
B. Protozoan infection
C. Blastomycosis
D. Mucormycosis
E. Sporotrichosis

220.

A 30-year-old woman lives in Houston, TX. She frequently buys fresh produce at a local stand set up by immigrant workers from the area south of Houston. She likes the selection and the prices are very good compared to supermarket prices. Unfortunately, after eating one of these selections, she develops severe diarrhea as does her family of 7. A strange organism called *Cyclospora* is diagnosed by her internist.

Based on this history, which of the following is the likely source for the *Cyclospora*?

A. Green beans
B. Raspberries
C. Fresh chicken
D. Milk
E. Her cat

221.

A 27-year-old Med-Peds resident travels frequently and asks about going to Southeast Asia for a mission trip and wonders about prophylaxis for various diseases.

Which of the following should he take for malaria prophylaxis?

   A. Chloroquine
   B. Chloroquine followed by primaquine
   C. Primaquine
   D. Atovaquone/proguanil followed by primaquine
   E. Quinine and clindamycin

222.

A 40-year-old man with AML is admitted with fever. His WBC count is 900 with 10% neutrophils. He is begun on cefepime. He is stable but continues to have fever; his ANC today (hospital day 7) is 40.

Which of the following agents would you start now?

   A. Add ciprofloxacin to the cefepime.
   B. Add vancomycin to the cefepime.
   C. Stop the cefepime and observe off antibiotics.
   D. Add liposomal amphotericin B to the cefepime.
   E. Do nothing new, just continue the cefepime.

223.

A nurse on the HIV unit of the local hospital presents to your employee health department. Today he is drawing blood on a patient with HIV and accidentally sticks himself with the needle he used to draw the blood. He quickly washes the hand thoroughly and reports to employee health.

Which of the following should happen next?

   A. Draw viral loads on the patient and, if undetectable, start Combivir® only.
   B. Begin interferon alpha-ribavirin.
   C. Start ZDV, 3TC, lopinavir/ritonavir.
   D. Start zidovudine only.
   E. No therapy is needed if he washed his hands well.

224.

A 30-year-old former IV drug user had a prosthetic aortic valve placed 1 month ago. He woke up yesterday with fever and chills and decided to come to see you today because the fever has persisted. He notes no other findings. Your physical examination at this point shows Janeway lesions. Blood cultures are drawn.

Based on his history, what is the likely etiology of his endocarditis?

A. *Staphylococcus aureus*, methicillin-sensitive
B. *Staphylococcus aureus*, methicillin-resistant
C. *Staphylococcus epidermidis*, methicillin-sensitive
D. *Staphylococcus epidermidis*, methicillin-resistant
E. Viridans streptococci

225.

A 40-year-old woman from Rhode Island presents to you with an isolated Bell's palsy. She awakened yesterday with this and now reports the weakness. She denies fever, headache, or other problems associated with this. She denies history of rash. She frequently goes hiking in the rural neighboring states but denies tick bite or other abnormality.

Based on this, which of the following is the most likely etiology for her palsy?

A. Multiple sclerosis
B. Lyme disease
C. Group A streptococcus immune response
D. Parvovirus B-19
E. Illicit Botox® use

226.

A 25-year-old man develops diarrhea after traveling to a water park in Georgia. He ate hamburgers and played in the "kiddie" pool while there. His diarrhea became bloody this morning, and he presents with fever and bloody stool. He has noted some abdominal cramping also. His physical examination is unremarkable except for a grossly positive heme on his rectal examination.

Cultures are sent and reveal enterohemorrhagic *E. coli.*

Based on this finding, which of the following antibiotics should you start?

A. Ciprofloxacin
B. Amoxicillin
C. Metronidazole
D. Clindamycin
E. No antibiotics

227.

A 35-year-old woman with AIDS (CD4 count 5) presents for evaluation. She has had HIV infection for 13 years and has done well on HAART therapy. She takes trimethoprim/sulfamethoxazole for PCP prophylaxis as well as azithromycin for MAC prophylaxis.

She presents today with worsening headache and vomiting. She has had low-grade temperatures for about a week. She denies vision changes.

Physical Examination:
HEENT: PERRLA, EOMI
TMs: Clear
Throat: Clear
Neck: ? meningismus
Heart: RRR with II/VI systolic flow murmur
Lungs: Few scattered crackles; cleared with coughing
Abdomen: + BS, soft, no hepatosplenomegaly
Extremities: No rashes noted

CT scan of the head with and without contrast: Normal; no evidence of increased intracranial pressure or lesions

CBC: WBC 2,500 with 50% lymphocytes
Hemoglobin: 11 mg/dL
Platelets: 225,000
Serum VDRL: Negative

Lumbar Puncture:
WBC 2 (100% lymphocytes)
CSF Protein 100 mg/dL (normal 30–80 mg/dL)
CSF Glucose 70 mg/dL (normal 60–90 mg/dL)

Gram stain: Negative
CSF VDRL: Negative

Based on the above results, which of the following do you recommend at this point?

   A. Begin empiric vancomycin and ceftriaxone.
   B. Begin ceftriaxone alone since the Gram stain is negative and pneumococcus is much less likely.
   C. Do a CSF antigen test for a fungus.
   D. Start IV penicillin 3 million units q 4 hours.
   E. Begin empiric INH/rifampin/ethambutol/PZA.

228.

An 80-year-old man lives in a nursing home. He has been hospitalized three times in the last 3 years for urosepsis. He has been forced to use a chronic indwelling catheter for incontinence after prostate surgery. He presents today with fever to 103° F and flank pain. He has chills and appears to be quite ill.
In the past he has had MRSA, *Enterococcus*, and *Pseudomonas* as a cause of his urosepsis.

What therapy do you recommend at this time?

   A. None, as this is likely just colonization.
   B. Ceftriaxone and gentamicin.
   C. Vancomycin and ceftazidime.
   D. Ciprofloxacin alone until sensitivities come back.
   E. Vancomycin and ceftriaxone.

229.

A 70-year-old woman is visiting the beautiful countryside of Colorado. She decides to take off her tennis shoes and goes walking in a field. While walking she steps on a dirty nail. She cries in pain and hobbles to a nearby meadow to sit down. While hobbling she steps in a huge cow patty. After sitting down her dog licks the injured foot. She comes into the Emergency Department wondering if she needs to have a tetanus immunization.

On history you learn she has had > 3 tetanus immunizations in the past, with the most recent 4 years ago.

What do you recommend for her besides avoiding nails, cow poop, and dogs licking her feet?

    A. She requires Td only.
    B. She requires Td and tetanus immune globulin.
    C. She requires tetanus immune globulin only.
    D. Wait and see if the wound becomes infected and then give Td.
    E. She requires no tetanus immunizations today.

230.

You are heading home from your long and grueling ABIM exam (which turned out to be quite easy, thanks to MedStudy), and you come across a woman at the local fast food hamburger store. She says her head hurts really badly. She is in line in front of you ordering 6 double burgers and mourning the death of Dave Thomas, the founder of Wendy's. Her boyfriend says that she has not been herself since about 3 hours ago. She has had fever to 102° F and says that she had a "drooping of her left face." She now complains of double vision.

You immediately have her transferred to the local hospital where you recommend which of the following to the nurse at the front desk?

    A. Admit this patient to psychiatry and order a lipid profile
    B. Get a STAT CT scan, then do a lumbar puncture, then give antibiotics if indicated
    C. Give intravenous antibiotics followed by a lumbar puncture
    D. Give oral antibiotics, then do a CT scan, then do a lumbar puncture if safe
    E. Give the patient intravenous antibiotics, then do a CT scan, and then do a lumbar puncture if safe

231.

A 40-year-old woman is receiving chemotherapy with cytarabine and daunorubicin for AML. She presents to the ED with a one-day history of intermittent chills and fever. She is noted to have a temperature of 103° F in the ED, and you are called immediately. Her physical examination is completely normal except for mucositis, some pallor, and tachycardia. She appears well otherwise. Laboratory studies reveal a WBC of 0.6 without neutrophils or bands. CXR and urinalysis are normal. Blood and urine cultures are taken.

Which of the following antibiotic choices is appropriate at this point?

    A. Ciprofloxacin and piperacillin/tazobactam
    B. Ceftriaxone and ampicillin
    C. Ceftriaxone and trimethoprim/sulfamethoxazole
    D. Vancomycin and ceftriaxone
    E. Vancomycin and cefepime

232.

Marla is a 28-year-old woman who steps on a dirty nail in a cow pasture. Her pet iguana licks the wound. Her last tetanus immunization (Td) was 6 years ago. Before that she received the usual immunization regiment as a child.

Which of the following does Marla require today?

A. Td only
B. Tdap only
C. Td and tetanus immune globulin
D. Tdap and tetanus immune globulin
E. DTaP and tetanus immune globulin

233.

An 18-year-old boy from Michigan presents for evaluation. Four days ago he stepped on a nail while wearing his tennis shoes. When this occurred, he was running in a cross country race in pastureland. The nail penetrated his tennis shoe and punctured his right foot. After the initial pain, he was fine. Last night however, he developed severe pain and swelling. Since last evening, he has been unable to bear weight on his foot. He is admitted to the hospital and a culture is obtained in the operating room.

The Gram stain shows gram-negative rods.

Based on this, which of the following is the most likely organism?

A. *E. coli*, if cows were in the pastureland he ran in
B. Leptospirosis
C. Group A streptococcus
D. *Pseudomonas aeruginosa*
E. Lyme disease

234.

A 40-year-old man with negative past medical history presents with a 1-week history of pain in his knees, wrists, and hands. He has been afebrile and has not had a rash. He lives in Massachusetts. Recently his 12-year-old daughter had an erythematous rash on her face (particularly her cheeks) and arms. Her rash got worse if she took a warm bath or was out in the sun. She also was afebrile.
His physical examination: Essentially normal except for his wrists and hands, which are moderately tender. No effusions of the joints are noted. He has no conjunctivitis or scleral changes on examination.

Which of the following is the likely etiology?

A. Human herpesvirus 6
B. Measles
C. *Borrelia burgdorferi*
D. Parvovirus B19
E. *Neisseria gonorrhoeae*

235.

A 52-year-old man is being evaluated because of a one-week history of lower extremity weakness, new onset of difficulty speaking, and decreased attention span (no jokes from the women out there about "how would a man know if he had a decreased attention span?"). He has had occasional diarrhea and abdominal pain in the last year. Of significance is that he has lost about 25 lbs during the past year. He complains of joint pains, particularly in his knees. He has had low-grade fever but no chills during the last year. He reports occasional night sweats. He has noted no other neurologic findings like seizures. His wife reports that areas of his skin are becoming darker—particularly those exposed to light.

Past Medical History: Healthy before this
Social History: Lives in Florida
                    Works as a bouncer for a teen-club
Family History: Negative

Physical Examination:
BP 130/80; T 99.9; P 84; RR 18
General: Alert, but oriented only to person and place!
HEENT: PERRLA, EOMI
Mild facial droop
Throat: Clear
Neck: Scattered lymphadenopathy in the anterior and posterior cervical chains; most nodes are 1x1 cm but a few are 2x1 cm
Heart: RRR without murmurs, rubs, and gallops
Lungs: CTA
Abdomen: Spleen tip palpated; no hepatomegaly;
A questionable abdominal mass discerned with deep palpation
Extremities: No cyanosis, clubbing, or edema
Neuro: Right lower extremity with increased tone and 4/5 muscle strength
Sensation is normal
Deep tendon reflexes are symmetrical

Laboratory:
Hemoglobin: 16.0 g/dL; Hematocrit: 52%
WBC: 29,000/mm^3; 65% neutrophils, 28% lymphs
ESR: 13 mm/hr
Glucose 200 mg/dL
Albumin 3.7 g/dL
ALT 32 U/L; AST 23 U/L
CT of the head shows a hypodense left frontal lobe lesion. A stereotactic brain biopsy is taken and shows acute inflammation and necrosis with <u>no</u> malignant cells. Gram stain shows 1+ WBCs but <u>no</u> organisms. However: A specimen stained with periodic acid-Schiff (PAS) shows multiple PAS-positive foamy macrophages.

Which of the following organisms is likely responsible for his condition?

    A. *Coxiella burnetii*
    B. *Mycobacterium tuberculosis*
    C. *Trophermyma whippleii*
    D. *Nocardia asteroides*
    E. *Actinomyces israelii*

236.

Which of the following infections or biological agents would prevent a mother from breast-feeding her baby for a period of time?

A. Received rubella vaccine today
B. Active, untreated tuberculosis
C. Received measles vaccine today
D. Received mumps vaccine today
E. Acute rubella infection

237.

A 22-year-old pop singer has been ill with diarrhea for the past 2 weeks. She says that she noted this while she was performing in Latin America. You are the physician for the cruise line that she is performing for now.

She tells you that she has had some low-grade temperatures since returning from her tour. She did not eat any fresh vegetables (unless you call French fries a fresh vegetable). She likes to eat beef jerky and prefers the "extra salty" version. She drank only bottled water and a soft drink for which she is a national spokesperson. She did drink these beverages poured over ice, but she thought that the "frozen stuff would kill the cooties."
She has not noted any blood in her stool. She has lost about 2 pounds in the last week.

Past Medical History: Cosmetic surgery at age 16
    Depression since age 14, on no medications at the moment

Social History: Sexually active with multiple partners
    Smokes 1 pack/day for the past 3 years
    Denies illicit drug use
    Denies use of alcohol

Family History: She and her mother are estranged at the moment
    Father left when she was 12 years of age
    Sister healthy
    Recently was married in Las Vegas; marriage was annulled after 24 hours—"I don't know what I was thinking."

Review of Systems: Diarrhea is intermittent, and she has crampy abdominal pain on occasion
    No rash
    No burning on urination
    No chills
    Diminished appetite

Physical Examination:
General: Pink hair with numerous piercings
VS: Temp 100.0° F, BP 110/70, Pulse 95, RR 16
HEENT: PERRLA, EOMI
Throat: Clear
Heart: RRR with no murmurs, rubs, or gallops
Lungs: CTA
Abd: Hyperactive bowel sounds, non-tender examination; no hepatosplenomegaly

GU: Normal female genitalia; no tenderness on bi manual palpation; no discharge noted
Extremities: No cyanosis, clubbing, or edema
Rectal: Heme positive (slight)

Laboratory:
Check for stool leukocytes: Positive
Giardia specific antigen: Negative
Stool culture: *Salmonella enteritidis* beta-lactamase producing

Based on this information, which of the following is the best treatment?

    A. Ciprofloxacin 500 mg bid for 10 days
    B. Erythromycin 500 mg bid for 5 days
    C. Tetracycline 500 mg qid for 10 days
    D. Amoxicillin 500 mg tid for 10 days
    E. No antibiotic therapy

NEPHROLOGY

238.

A 24-year-old Caucasian female was admitted to the hospital with progressive obtundation over a two-day period. She has a history of Crohn disease and has been taking monthly B_{12} injections since she had surgery two years earlier. A similar episode occurred one year earlier, and she improved shortly after admission. On physical exam her vital signs were: BP 112/66, P 88/min, R 22, T afebrile. She is a thin, obtunded woman, but arousable. Her exam was unremarkable except for a midline abdominal surgical scar, and she had no focal neurologic deficits.

Laboratory:
Hgb 11.6
HCT 34.1%
WBC 9,300
Na 136
K 3.1
Cl 90
CO_2 15
Glu 104
BUN 12
Cr 0.7
ABG: pH 7.22, pO_2 96, pCO_2 30, HCO_3 14.
She does not have an osmolar gap.

Which of the following is the most likely cause of her acidosis?

A. Ethylene glycol intoxication
B. D-lactic acidosis
C. Starvation ketosis
D. Lactic acidosis

239.

A 62-year-old man is brought to the hospital by ambulance acutely ill. He developed nausea, diarrhea, and a low-grade fever two days ago—and then developed progressive severe abdominal pain over the past 12 hours, which is so severe that he can hardly move. His past medical history is significant for glaucoma, for which he takes acetazolamide 250 mg tid, and a hospitalization for diverticulitis one year earlier. He does not have diabetes or hypertension.

Physical Exam: Appears extremely ill. BP 88/62, P 122, R 24, T 38.7° C (101.6° F).
His neck veins are not visible, even when he is supine
Heart and lungs are clear
Abdomen has absent bowel sounds with generalized rebound

Laboratory:
Hgb 13.1
HCT 39.6%
WBC 22,300
Na 144

K 3.2
Cl 112
CO_2 10
Glu 108
BUN 36
Scr 1.4
U/A: pH 5, Sp Gr 1.010, prot 1+, 2–4 hyaline casts.

CXR nl
Upright Abd: Air under diaphragm.
ABGs: pH 7.16, pO_2 94, pCO_2 24, HCO_3 10.
Emergency surgical consultation is obtained.

His acid-base diagnosis is which of the following?

A. Mixed anion gap acidosis and non-anion gap acidosis
B. Mixed anion gap acidosis and respiratory alkalosis
C. Mixed metabolic and respiratory acidosis
D. Mixed non-anion gap acidosis and metabolic alkalosis

240.

A 60-year-old man has advanced chronic kidney disease due to obstructive uropathy and recurrent UTIs. He continues to have recurrent infections and was hospitalized last month with an *E. coli* pyelonephritis. He has refused surgery offered to correct his BPH. He now takes a daily dose of trimethoprim/sulfamethoxazole as UTI prophylaxis. On physical exam, you note mild hypertension but no other significant findings. His nephrologist, who saw him last week, has not referred him for transplantation but feels he will need dialysis in less than 6 months.

Which of the following reasons would explain a delay in transplantation in this man?

A. He is too old.
B. He has recurrent infections.
C. He must not be on TMP/SMX within 12 months of a transplant.
D. He is ineligible for transplant because of his hypertension.
E. He must be on dialysis before getting a transplant.

241.

A 62-year-old man is seen for evaluation of severe back pain after coughing vigorously. In the Emergency Department, he has a pathologic compression fracture of T6. Laboratory studies demonstrate:
Hgb 8.7, HCT 38.7%, WBC 6,200, Na 135, K 2.9, Cl 106, CO_2 20, Glu 88,
BUN 14, Cr 1.3, Ca 11.1, Phos 1.4, Uric Acid 1.5, Alb 3.7.

U/A: pH 7.0, Sp. Gr. 1.008, blood negative, glu (3+).

This patient most likely has which of the following?

    A. Liddle syndrome
    B. Bartter syndrome
    C. Fanconi syndrome
    D. Gitelman syndrome
    E. Alport's syndrome

242.

A 36-year-old African-American male corporate attorney is seen for evaluation of asymptomatic hypertension. His mother and uncle are both hypertensive. PE: BP 164/110, P 84, R 12. In general he is athletic, slender, and his examination is normal. Labs: CBC, Electrolytes, and Biochem profile are normal except BUN 24, Cr 2.8. Urinalysis: pH 5.5, Specific Gravity 1.008, protein 4+, blood –, no cells or casts. Serologic studies are negative. Protein:creatinine ratio is 11.5. His renal biopsy is shown in Figure 1 (see color photos in back of book).

The most appropriate initial agent for treatment of his hypertension is which of the following?

    A. Angiotensin-converting enzyme inhibitor
    B. Thiazide diuretic
    C. Central alpha agonist
    D. Dihydropyridine calcium-channel blocker
    E. Beta-blocker

243.

A 62-year-old man is evaluated for renal failure. He had a 16-year history of hypertension, 15-year history of Type II diabetes, and still smokes 2 packs/day. Fourteen days earlier, he presented with abdominal pain, radiating to the back. On admission, his Hgb was 10.4, Cr was 1.3, and urinalysis negative. An aortogram confirmed an 8-cm abdominal aortic aneurysm, and he immediately went for surgical repair. He did very well and was discharged five days post-operatively with a Cr of 1.2 on HCTZ 12.5 mg/d, metoprolol 50 mg bid, and lisinopril 10 mg/d. He now returns because he has been running a fever and has a new rash on his feet.

Physical Exam:
BP 144/84, P 64, R 13, T 38.1° C (100.6° F). His surgical site is well healed and his examination is remarkable for blue discoloration of his toes as shown in Figure 2. (See photos in back of book.)

Laboratory: Hgb 10.9, HCT 34.1%, WBC 12,200 (12% eosinophils), Electrolytes normal, BUN 55, Cr 3.6. ESR 66, C3 55 (nl 70–110).

U/A: Sp Gr 1.008, pH 6, 1+ prot, 1+ blood, 2–5 RBCs/HPF, 2–4 hyaline casts.

The most likely cause of his acute renal failure is which of the following?

    A. Endocarditis-associated glomerulonephritis
    B. Systemic vasculitis
    C. Radiocontrast-induced acute renal failure
    D. Renal artery embolization
    E. Cholesterol atheroembolic disease

244.

A 25-year-old girl begins to experience recurrent headaches at the start of a new job on Wall Street as a stock analyst. Her work performance has been excellent, her menses are regular and not associated with many of these headaches, and she takes no over-the-counter medications or prescription drugs. She does have a family history of hypertension and Type 2 diabetes mellitus. On physical, her BP is 188/110 (her records indicate she has had a normal BP on prior visits). She is tall and thin, and she has symmetric and strong pulses. Her cardiovascular exam is otherwise normal with the exception of a faint diastolic bruit to the right of her umbilicus. Her lungs are clear; she has an otherwise unremarkable exam.

Which of the following diagnoses is most likely at this point?

    A. Coarctation of the aorta
    B. Essential hypertension
    C. Cocaine use
    D. Stress of the new job and economic meltdown
    E. Fibromuscular dysplasia

245.

Which of the following is a usual feature of acute renal failure caused by intravenous contrast?

    A. Oliguria
    B. Irreversible
    C. Uncommon in diabetics
    D. May be prevented with increased hydration before the procedure
    E. Rare in multiple myeloma patients

246.

A 45-year-old woman has been on hemodialysis for two years and has recently been activated on the transplant waiting list. Her current medications are atenolol 50 mg/d, multivitamin with B, C, and folic acid qd, erythropoietin 4,000 subcutaneous once a week, and calcium carbonate 1,000 mg tid. Routine screening studies reveal the following laboratory findings: Ca 9.9 (nl: 8.5–10.4), Phos 5.2 (nl: 2.5–3.9), Alb 4.1 (nl: 3.5–4.9), intact PTH level: 646 (nl: 75–110).

What would be the appropriate management of her elevated PTH level?

    A. Add a vitamin D analog.
    B. No change in her therapy is necessary at this time.
    C. Add sevelamer (Renagel®).
    D. Refer for parathyroidectomy.
    E. Increase the calcium carbonate to 1,500 mg tid.

247.

A 72-year-old African-American patient with a 15-year history of hypertension and 6-year history of Type 2 DM is referred for evaluation of renal disease. Over the past 5 years, his creatinine has been slowly increasing. He had a partial colectomy 6 months ago for colon cancer. At this visit his blood pressure is 150/90, funduscopic exam shows AV nicking, and cardiac exam shows the PMI is displaced. Medications: enalapril 20 mg/bid, glyburide 5 mg/daily, and furosemide 20 mg/daily.

Laboratory: Hgb 11 g/dL, Na 145 mEq/L, Cl 10 mEq/L, K 4.7 mEq/L, CO_2 20 mEq/L, Glu 146, BUN 48 mg/dL, and Cr 4.3 mg/dL.
U/A: 4+ protein, no blood, microscopic exam is negative.

Which of the following should you do now?

A. Obtain serum and urine Na and Cr to calculate fractional sodium excretion for prerenal azotemia.
B. Arrange for a temporary dialysis catheter so that he can start dialysis within the next week.
C. Refer to your vascular surgeon for native AV fistula construction.
D. Refer for transplant evaluation and listing.

248.

A 24-year-old Caucasian man is referred to you for evaluation of microscopic hematuria found on a pre-employment physical examination. His history reveals no recent respiratory or skin infections, no urinary tract symptoms, and no family history of renal disease. On physical examination his BP was 130/84 mmHg with no other abnormalities. His CBC, biochem profile, and electrolytes are normal. Serologies for hepatitis B and C are negative. Complement levels are normal. His Cr = 1.8 mg/dL, U/A by you reveals: Sp Gr 1.016, 2+ blood, 2+ protein, negative glucose, 20–30 "dysmorphic" RBCs/HPF, 0–2 WBCs/HPF, 5–10 RBC casts/LPF, and 2–3 granular casts/LPF.

Given this information, which of the following is his most likely diagnosis?

A. Membranoproliferative glomerulonephritis
B. IgA nephropathy
C. Systemic lupus erythematosus
D. Membranous glomerulonephritis
E. Minimal change disease

249.

A 20-year-old Vietnamese immigrant comes to your office complaining of ankle edema of one-week duration. His history reveals no other medical problems, and his physical examination is normal except for pitting edema that extends to his thighs. Cr is 0.7 mg/dL. Serum albumin is 0.9. Protein:Creatinine ratio is16.5. U/A: Sp Gr 1.020, 4+ protein, negative blood, negative glucose, 0–2 RBCs/HPF, 0–2 WBCs/HPF, 2+ oval fat bodies and 5–10 hyaline casts/LPF. Serologic studies are normal.

The most appropriate initial therapy would be which of the following?

    A. Azathioprine 2 mg/kg/d
    B. Methylprednisolone 1 gm qd x 3
    C. Cyclophosphamide 500 mg/m^2
    D. Prednisone 1 mg/kg/d
    E. Cyclosporine 5 mg/kg/dL

250.

A previously healthy 45-year-old woman is admitted with severe diarrhea. Her physical exam is notable for very dry mucosa and a SBP in the low 80s. Her abdomen is diffusely tender, but her physical exam is otherwise unremarkable. Her labs are generally normal, with the exception of a creatinine of 1.8 mg/dL and a urine SG of 1.030 (with an otherwise bland U/A). In addition, you obtain urinary studies and estimate a fractional excretion of sodium (FENa) of less than 1%.

What diagnosis does this constellation support?

    A. HUS/TTP
    B. Prerenal azotemia
    C. Acute tubular necrosis
    D. Acute rejection
    E. Goodpasture syndrome

251.

A 65-year-old man with a long-standing history of hypertension, previous coronary artery bypass grafting, fem-pop bypass, and CHF is seen for new-onset hip pain, presumed secondary to osteoarthritis. His current medications are metoprolol 25 mg bid, hydrochlorothiazide 25 mg daily, ASA 81 mg/d, and lisinopril 20 mg/day. Baseline labs include a serum creatinine of 1.8 mg/day and normal electrolytes and urinalysis. He is given a prescription for ibuprofen 600 mg tid. He returns five days later complaining of edema. Repeat labs: Serum creatinine 2.8, potassium 6.2; urinalysis is normal.

The most likely cause for his change in renal function is which of the following?

    A. Acute tubular necrosis secondary to ibuprofen
    B. Acute interstitial nephritis secondary to ibuprofen
    C. Prerenal azotemia secondary to ibuprofen
    D. Acute papillary necrosis secondary to ibuprofen
    E. Acute glomerulonephritis secondary to ibuprofen

252.

A 57-year-old normotensive woman with a 14-year history of Type 2 diabetes is found to have microalbuminuria and is started on losartan 50 mg daily. On follow-up, her creatinine has not changed, but her potassium is now 6.5.

Which of the following is the most likely mechanism for hyperkalemia when losartan is added?

A. The patient has an underlying Type II RTA.
B. The patient has an underlying Type IV RTA.
C. The patient has an underlying Type I RTA.
D. The patient has underlying obstructive uropathy.
E. The patient has underlying Gitelman syndrome.

253.

Which of the following is <u>true</u> with regard to arterial blood gases?

A. There is no full compensation for primary acid-base disorders.
B. The generation of an anion gap is physiologically unlimited.
C. 1 mmol of generated acid may result in more than 1 mmol of bicarbonate.
D. All anions are accounted for in routine blood chemistries.
E. All of the answer options are false.

254.

A 32-year-old woman presents with the following laboratory values: Na 140, K 2.8, Cl 113, CO_2 15, BUN 12, Cr 1.1.

U/A: pH 6.5, no blood, protein, or casts. ABGs: pH 7.34, pCO_2 31, HCO_3 16. Urine Na 65, Urine K 8, Urine Cl 94.

Which of the following is the most likely diagnosis?

A. Laxative abuse
B. Surreptitious vomiting
C. Type I RTA
D. Type II RTA
E. Type IV RTA

255.

A previously healthy 82-year-old woman with "bad knees" is brought to the Emergency Department by her family with mental obtundation. She has no focal findings. Her laboratory studies reveal the following: Na 140, Cl 101, K 3.9, CO_2 12, glucose-normal, Cr 1.4.
U/A normal.
ABGs: pH 7.25, pO_2 97, pCO_2 22, HCO_3 12.

Which of the following is the most likely diagnosis?

A. Ethylene glycol intoxication
B. Type I RTA
C. D-lactic acidosis
D. Salicylate intoxication
E. Starvation ketosis

256.

A 25-year-old man presents with hematuria and a serum creatinine of 1.6. An ultrasound demonstrates numerous cysts in both kidneys. The patient's father is a renal transplant recipient, as are numerous other relatives. While he has not had any headaches, he asks you about the association of cerebral aneurysms with polycystic kidney disease and wonders if he needs a CT scan of his head.

Which of the following do you recommend?

    A. Order a CT scan of the head to screen for aneurysms.
    B. Order no tests.
    C. Order an MRI of the head to screen for aneurysms.
    D. Perform cerebral angiography.
    E. Order molecular screening for the polycystic kidney disease (PCKD) gene.

257.

An obese, 37-year-old woman has been recently diagnosed with diabetes mellitus Type 2. You spend considerable time discussing weight loss, proper eating, and a healthy lifestyle.

To screen for microvascular disease and kidney disease in particular, which of the following is appropriate?

    A. Screen for microalbuminuria now.
    B. Wait 5 years before screening for microalbuminuria.
    C. The standard urine dipstick is sufficient for screening for diabetic kidney disease.
    D. Focus on weight loss and deal with the kidneys later.
    E. An eye exam will suffice to check for all microvascular disease.

258.

Which of the following is the most likely set of electrolytes for a healthy 48-year-old man as he crosses the finish line of a 10K road race in New Orleans in July (average temp 92° F, average humidity 98%)?

    A. Serum Na 125, Cl 90, K 3.9, CO_2 26, Urine osm 950
    B. Serum Na 155, Cl 118, K 3.9, CO_2 26, Urine osm 150
    C. Serum Na 155, Cl 120, K 3.9, CO_2 22, Urine osm 950
    D. Serum Na 155, Cl 118, K 3.9, CO_2 26, Urine osm 950
    E. Serum Na 125, Cl 90, K 3.9, CO_2 26, Urine osm 150

259.

You are asked to evaluate a 66-year-old man with cirrhosis for acute renal failure because, over the last week, his urine output has fallen and his BUN and Cr have risen to 40 and 4.2, respectively. He was admitted to the hospital 7 days earlier with spontaneous bacterial peritonitis, and therapy was initiated with ceftazidime and vancomycin; abdominal pain has been slowly improving.

Physical Examination:
BP 114/74, P 80, afebrile. In general, he is a chronically ill gentleman without jaundice.
His central venous pressure is 9 cm
Heart and lungs are normal
Moderate ascites, without abdominal tenderness
There is 1+ peripheral edema.

Laboratory:
Na 133
K 4.1
Cl 98
CO_2 22
BUN 40
Cr 4.2
Urinalysis: Specific gravity 1.007, pH 5.5, trace-protein, no blood, 1+ UBG, 2–5 RBCs/HPF, no WBCs, 4–6 granular casts/LPF. Fractional excretion of Na is 3.2%.
Ultrasound of the kidneys is normal.

The most likely cause of his acute renal failure is which of the following?

A. Acute interstitial nephritis
B. Hepatorenal syndrome
C. Acute tubular necrosis
D. Prerenal azotemia
E. Non-dilated obstructive uropathy

260.

A 27-year-old woman with focal segmental glomerulosclerosis is seen for a scheduled follow-up visit. She has no complaints. Her BP is 123/76; the remainder of the exam is normal. Meds: furosemide
40 mg bid and lisinopril 20 mg daily.

Labs: Na 138, K 4.1, Cl 101, CO_2 24, Glu 96, Hgb 9.5, HCT 28.7%, WBC 6,700, serum creatinine 3.5 mg/dL (unchanged from 3 months earlier). U/A: Sp Gr 1.003, pH 5.5, prot 1+, blood (–), no cells or casts.

What would be most appropriate to do at this visit?

A. Measure serum iron saturation and ferritin levels.
B. Discontinue lisinopril.
C. Discontinue furosemide.
D. Measure serum erythropoietin levels.
E. Measure RBC folate and B_{12} levels.

261.

A 65-year-old woman is evaluated because of a serum creatinine of 4.4 mg/dL on a routine follow-up visit. At her last office visit 8 months ago, her Cr was 1.2 mg/dL. She has a 12-year history of hypertension, treated with hydrochlorothiazide (HCTZ) 25 mg/d. She denies any new symptoms, and her physical examination is unchanged. Laboratory studies: Na 135, K 3.8, Cl 104, CO_2 25, Glu 103, BUN 44, Cr 4.4. Hgb 8.3, HCT 24.9%, WBC 6.5, Ca 10.5, Phos 5.5, albumin 2.8.

U/A: SpGr 1.004, pH 6, protein 3+, blood (–), no cells or casts.

The most likely diagnosis is which of the following?

A. Minimal change disease
B. Multiple myeloma
C. Membranoproliferative glomerulonephritis
D. Focal segmental glomerulosclerosis
E. IgA nephropathy

262.

Which of the following statements about aminoglycoside associated nephrotoxicity is <u>true</u>?

A. There typically is a lag time of 7–10 days after the start of therapy before clinical evidence of ATN (acute tubular necrosis) begins to occur.
B. Nephrotoxicity is not proportionate to the total dose of aminoglycoside.
C. Other nephrotoxic agents decrease the risk of ATN.
D. Co-administration of dopamine reduces the risk.
E. Elevated trough levels decrease the risk of ATN.

263.

Justin Frank is a 24-year-old man brought in by ambulance after being shot in an altercation at a local strip club. He arrives with a blood pressure of 80/30, with bleeding exit wounds at his chest and neck.

Laboratory:
Hemoglobin: 8.9 mg/dL, Hematocrit 24%

Na	139
K	3.9
Cl	101
HCO_3	10
pH	7.10
pCO_2	26
HCO_3	12

What is the acid-base diagnosis?

A. Primary metabolic alkalosis only
B. Primary metabolic acidosis only
C. Primary metabolic acidosis with secondary respiratory alkalosis
D. Primary metabolic alkalosis with secondary respiratory acidosis
E. Primary metabolic acidosis with secondary metabolic acidosis

264.

Mark Perkins is an 18-year-old referred to you for routine care from his pediatrician. He has a history of hematuria, which his uncle and brothers also have. No women in his family have this disorder. He also has nerve deafness.

Which of the following disorders is most likely?

A. Polyarteritis nodosa
B. Berger disease
C. Alport syndrome
D. Bloom syndrome
E. X-linked hematuria syndrome

265.

A 35-year-old African-American man presents with colicky abdominal pain. It is particularly bad in his left flank. He has no prior history of this type of pain. His father has a history of kidney stones. He has low-grade fevers and has vomited a few times this morning.

Plain x-ray of the abdomen done in the ED shows a radiodense area in the left renal pelvis. He passes a stone the next day, and it is determined to be a calcium stone.

Which of the following is true?

A. He should decrease his daily water intake.
B. He should decrease his dietary intake of vegetables and fruit.
C. Hydrochlorothiazide would be useful in reducing his risk of stone formation.
D. Furosemide would be useful in reducing his risk of stone formation.
E. He should increase his dietary intake of sodium chloride.

266.

A 40-year-old man has had Crohn disease for 20 years. He has had all of the classic symptoms and signs. He seems to be well controlled with mesalamine. However, he has had bouts of steatorrhea fairly frequently. Today, he presents with new-onset colicky flank pain with fever. You suspect a kidney stone.

What is the most likely type of stone that he has?

A. Calcium struvite
B. Calcium oxalate
C. Calcium carbonate
D. Calcium chloride
E. Calcium budesonide

267.

A 20-year-old man is admitted with severe diarrhea and the following laboratory data:
Sodium 142 mEq/L
Potassium 3.6 mEq/L
Chloride 115 mEq/L
Bicarbonate 12 mEq/L
Creatinine 1.1 mg/dL
pH 7.12, PCO_2 38, HCO_3 12
(Normal Anion Gap for this lab is 4–16.)
Urine ketones: Negative

What acid-base disorders are present?

   A. Metabolic acidosis only
   B. Respiratory alkalosis and metabolic acidosis
   C. Normal anion gap metabolic acidosis and respiratory acidosis
   D. Normal anion gap metabolic acidosis and respiratory alkalosis
   E. High anion gap metabolic acidosis and respiratory acidosis

268.

A 19-year-old college student presents with complaints of blood in his urine. He states that it usually occurs after exercising, although he did notice that about one month ago when he had "a cold," he also had dark-colored urine. He has no other complaints and has been in good health. He has no allergies and doesn't take any medications. He denies use of alcohol or illicit drugs.

Physical Examination:
BP 120/70, P 60, RR 18, Temp 98.5° F
HEENT: WNL
Heart: RRR without murmurs, rubs, or gallops
Lungs: CTA
Abdomen: Normal bowel sounds, no hepatosplenomegaly
Extremities: No cyanosis, clubbing, or edema
Laboratory: U/A shows moderate RBCs with occasional RBC casts and occasional WBCs. He has no proteinuria. BUN 11 mg/dL, Creatinine 0.7 mg/dL. Complement levels are normal.

Which of the following is the likely diagnosis?

   A. Wegener granulomatosis
   B. Polyarteritis nodosa
   C. SLE
   D. IgA nephropathy
   E. Membranoproliferative glomerular nephritis

269.

A 28-year-old man with known autosomal dominant polycystic kidney disease (PKD) has had a first episode of bleeding and painful cyst. You have treated him as an inpatient with IV hydration and pain medications. Since he is a new transfer to your care, you counsel him that he may suffer a number of non-renal complications from his PKD.

Which of the following complications should you inform him of with regard to his PKD?

A. Diverticulosis.
B. Mitral valve prolapse.
C. Intracranial aneurysms.
D. Recurrent flank pain.
E. All of the answers are complications of PKD.

270.

A 16-year-old girl is brought to the ED by her mother, who reports that she is behaving strangely. She spent most of the day at home alone despite several invitations by friends to go out. You are unable to elicit additional information from the patient because she falls asleep each time you speak to her. She does have a history of depression and has seen a counselor for bulimia. She takes no medications. Her mother reports suspicions regarding use of both tobacco and alcohol. On physical exam, her blood pressure is 90/60 mmHg, pulse 115, and respirations 16. She is a thin, pale girl who is clearly obtunded. A funduscopic exam is normal. Her lungs are clear, heart sounds normal, and abdomen soft. Her lab work is notable for the following: Na 140, K 4.0, Cl 105, HCO_3 15, Glucose 98, Creatinine 0.8, and BUN 12. A U/A has a SG of 1.020, pH 5.2, and several urate crystals. A STAT drug and ethanol screen is negative. A measured serum osmolality is 345.

What is your provisional diagnosis?

A. Acute aspirin overdose
B. Binge eating with vomiting and dehydration
C. Anti-freeze ingestion
D. Non-ketotic hyperosmolar coma
E. Diabetic ketoacidosis

271.

A previously healthy 17-year-old boy is brought to you with tea-colored urine that was first noted today. He has a runny nose and cough (without fever) that started yesterday. A similar episode occurred once last winter and resolved after 3 days without intervention. You note in the chart 2 episodes of strep throat with positive strep screens that occurred 4 months ago and 6 months ago. His physical exam is entirely normal. A U/A confirms too-numerous-to-count RBCs and positive protein on a dipstick. An extensive lab exam shows a normal ASO, normal complement levels, and a normal creatinine.

Your leading diagnosis is which of the following?

A. Pseudohematuria
B. IgA nephropathy
C. Endocarditis
D. Post-streptococcal GN
E. Lupus nephritis

272.

A 15-year-old girl presents to the ED with bloody diarrhea. She attended a local county fair 3 days earlier. Her diarrhea started today, accompanied by crampy abdominal pain and fever to 102° F. She appears ill and sometimes confused. She has a BP of 175/110 mmHg and a pulse of 96. Her lungs have crackles one-third of the way up, and a loud 3/6 systolic murmur is audible. The abdominal exam is diffusely tender but lacks peritoneal signs. She has no edema. Her U/A has numerous RBCs and an occasional RBC cast. Her hematocrit is 18%, WBC 8,800 with 80% polys, and platelets 78,000. A stat BMP returns with a Na 122, K 6.2, Cl 98, HCO_3 18, Glucose 110, BUN 62, Creatinine 4.4, and Ca 8.8.

Which of the following would be the next step in confirming the diagnosis?

A. Measure complement, hepatis B and C serologies, liver function tests, ANCA, ANA, and anti-GBM antibodies.
B. Obtain a stat chest x-ray and blood gases.
C. Perform a rectal examination.
D. Review a peripheral smear for presence of schistocytes.
E. Order a stat renal ultrasound to exclude obstruction.

273.

A 23-year-old college student presents with a one-week history of swollen ankles and face. He has no previous medical history and is taking no medications. On physical examination, his vital signs are normal, and the only significant findings are 2–3+ swelling in his legs, up to his thighs.

Initial lab studies: CBC and electrolytes are normal, serum creatinine 0.9 mg/dL, BUN 11 mg/dL, serum albumin 1.1. Urinalysis has 4+ protein and oval fat bodies but no blood or casts. Urine protein:creatinine is 8.5.

Which of the following would you expect from this patient?

A. He is likely to respond to prednisone 1 mg/kg/day.
B. He is unlikely to respond to prednisone 1 mg/kg/day.
C. He is likely to develop progressive renal failure.
D. He should be treated with pulse methylprednisolone and chlorambucil.
E. He is likely to have low serum complements.

274.

A 74-year-old woman develops acute flank pain and comes to the Emergency Department. She has a history of hypertension as well as an MI five years earlier. She has never had any UTIs and denies dysuria.

Physical Exam:
BP 180/110, P 124, irregularly, irregular; T 38.5° C (101.3° F).
She is acutely ill and has right CVA tenderness.

ECG: Atrial fibrillation, rate 122–132, left axis deviation.

Laboratory:
WBC 23,500
Hgb 12.2
Serum creatinine 3.1
BUN 45
Urinalysis: 1+ protein, 3+ blood, 0–2 WBCs/HPF, 15–25 RBCs/HPF, 2–4 granular casts
CPK 201
LDH 7,100
Ultrasound of the kidneys: Kidneys 9.5 cm each, no obstruction

The most likely diagnosis is which of the following?

A. Renal artery embolization
B. Pyelonephritis
C. Acute papillary necrosis
D. Right nephrolithiasis
E. Ruptured renal cyst

275.

A 57-year-old man with known membranous nephropathy associated with 8.5 grams of proteinuria per day presents with increasing cough and shortness of breath, along with fever and malaise of 6-hours duration. He has a BP of 146/78, pulse 96, temp of 39° C (102.2° F) and O_2 saturation of 91% on room air. His physical exam is notable for a normal cardiac exam—except for a 2/6 systolic ejection murmur; wheezes and crackles at the bases of both lungs; a soft abdomen; and severe, lower-extremity edema but with no leg pain or tenderness. Initial labs are essentially normal except for an albumin of 2.5 mg/dL and an elevated WBC of 17,000. A standard ECG is normal.

Which study is most appropriate to perform next and is likely to confirm the diagnosis of the cause of his shortness of breath?

A. Duplex sonography of both lower extremities
B. Serial CK-MBs and troponins
C. Chest x-ray and sputum culture
D. CT angiography of the chest
E. Right-sided ECG

ENDOCRINOLOGY

276.

A patient of yours is a 35-year-old man who had a thyroid nodule that proved to be cancerous. After his thyroidectomy, the final pathology report mentioned a 4.2-cm mass containing a well-differentiated papillary cancer. There was no growth of the cancer into adjacent structures and no evidence of metastases into any lymph nodes. He received high-dose radioactive iodine ablation after surgery. His total body scan was negative, and he is now on a suppressive dose of thyroxine. He is in your office for a routine follow-up. He is clinically euthyroid, the TSH is 0.30 mU/L (0.5–5.0 mU/L), and the free-thyroxine (FT4) is 1.4 ng/dL (0.7–1.5 ng/dL).

He asks you about the risk of recurrence of his thyroid cancer.

Which of the following responses should you give him?

  A. There is no increased risk for recurrence.
  B. The risk for recurrence is increased due to his gender.
  C. The risk for recurrence is increased due to the type of cancer.
  D. The risk for recurrence is increased due to the size of the tumor.
  E. The risk for recurrence is increased due to his age.

277.

A 66-year-old woman recently diagnosed by her cardiologist 3 months ago with Type 2 diabetes mellitus is in your office for a routine follow-up. She also has stage III congestive heart failure, which is closely followed by her cardiologist, who recently placed a note in her chart stating that the CHF is currently stable. She follows an American Heart Association step 3 diet and a cardiologist-approved walking program as well as she can. She takes her prescription drugs exactly as instructed, including metformin 500 mg at bedtime. She steadfastly refuses to take insulin. Her glycemic control is less than desired. The fasting glucose levels average 90–100, postprandial levels 200–210, and bedtime levels 100–120. The HgbA1c is 8.2 %, serum creatinine is 1.4 mg/dL, AST/ALT are normal, and bilirubin is normal.

Which of the following should be used to improve her glycemic control?

  A. Increase metformin to 1,000 mg twice daily in steps as tolerated.
  B. Add pioglitazone 45 mg once daily or rosiglitazone 4 mg twice daily.
  C. Add acarbose 50 mg with every meal.
  D. Stop metformin and begin repaglinide 1 mg before meals.
  E. Stop metformin and begin either pioglitazone or rosiglitazone.

278.

A 24-year-old man with hypocalcemia is referred to you. He has a history of alcohol abuse and poor nutrition during his bouts of drinking. Prior episodes of hypomagnesemia were all related to bouts of alcohol abuse and spontaneously resolved within two weeks of abstinence. The patient's primary care provider noticed the hypocalcemia this time and has not been able to explain it. The patient reports fatigue and muscle cramps. You are not able to elicit Chvostek or Trousseau signs. You puzzle over the pertinent lab results until you realize the explanation for hypocalcemia is staring you in the face.

Na$^+$	140 mEq/L (135–143 mEq/L)
K$^+$	4.2 mEq/L (3.5–5.0 mEq/L)
Cl$^-$	104 mEq/L (100–109 mEq/L)
HCO$_3^-$	24 mEq/L (22–30 mEq/L)
Urea nitrogen	10 mg/dL (8–18 mg/dL)
Creatinine	0.8 mg/dL (0.6–1.2 mg/dL)
Glucose	88 mg/dL (65–110 mg/dL)
Albumin	4.5 g/dL (4.0–6.0 g/dL)
Ca^{+2}	7.9 mg/dL (8.5–10.5 mg/dL)
Phosphorus	4.9 mg/dL (1.5–4.5 mg/dL)
Mg^{+2}	0.5 mg/dL (1.4–2.5 mg/dL)

25(OH)-Vitamin D	40 µg/L (10–55 µg/L)
1,25(OH)$_2$-Vitamin D	13 ng/L (18–62 ng/L)
intact PTH	6 pg/mL (10–65 pg/mL).

As expected, all of the above labs normalize within one week of abstaining from alcohol and taking magnesium supplements.

What was the most likely cause of this patient's hypocalcemia?

    A. Pseudohypocalcemia
    B. Barter syndrome
    C. Hypoparathyroidism due to hypomagnesemia
    D. Pseudohypoparathyroidism
    E. Familial hypocalciuric hypocalcemia

279.

A 47-year-old man comes to see you after being told that he needs to see a physician. He is an admitted "health freak" and recently underwent a voluntary DXA scan for body composition determination. The test showed body fat content a little below average and a bone density that was 1.5 standard deviations below average for young men (Z-score –1.5).

The radiologist reviewing the test told him that his bones were less dense than they should be and that he should see a physician. In your office, he admits to taking mega-doses of vitamins but is unable to recall which ones. He reports some mild bone and muscle pain, which he attributes to his long workouts. Your examination fails to detect anything abnormal. His blood pressure is normal. Laboratory tests are as follows:

Na$^+$	140 mEq/L (135–143 mEq/L)
K$^+$	4.9 mEq/L (3.5–5.0 mEq/L)
Cl$^-$	104 mEq/L (100–109 mEq/L)
HCO$_3^-$	23 mEq/L (22–30 mEq/L)
Urea nitrogen	10 mg/dL (8–18 mg/dL)
Creatinine	0.8 mg/dL (0.6–1.2 mg/dL)
Glucose	88 mg/dL (65–110 mg/dL)
Albumin	4.5 g/dL (4.0–6.0 g/dL)
Ca^{+2}	10.9 mg/dL (8.5–10.5 mg/dL)
Phosphorus	5.2 mg/dL (1.5–4.5 mg/dL)

25(OH)-Vitamin D	63 µg/L (10–55 µg/L)
1,25(OH)$_2$-Vitamin D	19 ng/L (18–62 ng/L)
intact PTH	1 pg/mL (10–65 pg/mL)

Which of the following might explain his hypercalcemia and osteopenia?

A. Vitamin D intoxication
B. Excess calcium in his diet
C. Vitamin A intoxication
D. Surreptitious use of thiazide diuretics
E. Hypoparathyroidism

280.

A 21-year-old woman comes to see you in the university health clinic complaining of no menses for two months. She has been doing well in her studies and denies any unusual stress. On the contrary, she greatly enjoys the swim team and has been doing quite well lately. She reports that her menses began at age 13, and her periods have been regular as far back as she can remember. Her vital signs are BP 100/70 mmHg and pulse 65/min. Your examination reveals a well-developed female with no abnormalities that can be detected by your pelvic exam. She has no clitoromegaly, her breasts are at Tanner stage V, her pubic hair pattern is at Tanner stage IV, and nothing can be expressed from her breasts. You notice that she walks with a slight limp, which she attributes to an old ankle injury due to a boating accident and says it bothers her only during weight-bearing activities. A urine pregnancy test is negative, and she denies sexual activity since she broke up with her boyfriend 9 months ago. She was depressed at the time, but filled the void with more time in the pool. She denies any prescription or illicit drug use.

Which of the following causes of amenorrhea can be <u>eliminated</u> from the differential diagnosis?

A. Post-pill amenorrhea
B. Swimming-induced amenorrhea
C. A pituitary tumor
D. Congenital adrenal hyperplasia
E. Exogenous androgens

281.

A new patient comes to your office complaining of a lump in her neck. She is 18 years old and reports first noticing the lump 6 months ago. She delayed seeing you because she thought it would go away. She reports no change in size during the past 6 months and denies any problems with swallowing or breathing. There is no family history of thyroid disease, and she denies any exposure to radiation. Her voice is normal and the nodule is 3 cm, nontender, and movable. She does not exhibit any cervical lymphadenopathy. She is clinically euthyroid. You tell her that thyroid nodules are fairly common and thyroid cancer is relatively rare, but that you wish to begin a workup. She asks you if she has any increased risk for thyroid cancer.

Which of the following should be your response?

A. You must first check her TSH level.
B. You must first check her free T4 level.
C. She has no increased risk.
D. She has an increased risk because of her gender.
E. She has an increased risk because of her age.

282.

A 47-year-old woman comes to your clinic complaining of night sweats and marked mood swings. She says that she is experiencing the same unbearable symptoms of menopause that her mother experienced and she wants relief. She routinely exercises, and she has already tried the diet changes recommended in the lay press. She had a hysterectomy 20 years ago due to a complication of childbirth. There is no family history of breast cancer or thromboembolic disease. You agree with her that she is most likely experiencing marked symptoms of menopause. She asks about hormone replacement therapy because her mother got relief from it. You review the recent evidence against it and discuss other options with her, but she insists on trying hormones. You give her some literature, refer her for a mammogram, ask the lab to measure FSH, and schedule a follow-up appointment. The mammogram is negative, and the FSH confirms menopause. She still wants to try hormone therapy, so you start her on low-dose estrogen. She comes back in three months and reports feeling much better and thanks you for the estrogen. You remind her that hormone therapy can increase her risk of death, but she still wants the hormone therapy. It has been almost five years since you last checked her lipids, so you ask her to return in 3–4 months for fasting lipids. The HDL and non-HDL cholesterol are acceptable, but the triglycerides have markedly increased from 107 mg/dL to 820 mg/dL.

Which of the following should be done at this time?

A. Hold the estrogen and resume once the triglycerides are normal again.
B. Continue the estrogen and recheck lipids in 6–12 months.
C. Switch from estrogen to black cohosh from her local health food store.
D. Switch from oral estrogen to a transdermal patch.
E. Stop treating her symptoms despite her preferences.

283.

A 26-year-old woman comes to your clinic complaining of a neck mass. The mass does not hurt, but it has been present for 3 months without going away. In fact, she thinks it is now a little larger. She denies dysphagia, odynophagia, breathing difficulty, or changes in her voice. There is no history of exposure to radiation. She is afebrile and clinically euthyroid. The mass is a 1.8-cm nodule in the lower right pole of her thyroid gland. You order thyroid tests and have her return in one week for a fine needle biopsy. The TSH and FT4 are within normal limits. She returns in one week, and you inform her that she has medullary thyroid cancer. You schedule a thyroidectomy and post-surgical, high-dose radioactive iodine for ablation of any remnants. On further questioning, you learn that her mother died at age 39 from an unknown cause. She has two sisters, one brother, and a 2-year-old son.

Which laboratory test should be ordered to help assess the risk of her first-degree relatives developing medullary thyroid cancer?

A. Ret-proto-oncogene (*RET*)
B. Serum calcium
C. Serum gastrin
D. Serum calcium after administering gastrin
E. Serum calcium after administering calcitonin

284.

A new patient comes to your clinic for routine follow-up. He is 41 years old and has Type 2 diabetes. He reports fairly good compliance with diet and exercise. His BMI is 24.8 kg/m², and he briskly walks 3 miles every day after work. His last dilated eye exam was 6 months ago and no abnormalities were reported. He checks his capillary glucose levels once or twice a day, and his logbook shows reasonable glycemic control. He has a history of hyperlipidemia and is fully compliant with the diet recommended by a dietitian. He has tried and failed to tolerate niacin, bile acid sequestrants, and fibrates because of side effects. He also experienced hypersensitivity to ezetimibe. Your exam today is unremarkable, and his feet are okay. You order repeat fasting lipids and HbA1c. He comes back for follow-up of his lab tests, which are reported as follows:

HbA1c   6.9 %
ALT   120 IU/L (0–55 IU/L)
LDL   175 mg/dL
HDL   33 mg/dL
Triglycerides 127 mg/dL.

He denies any alcohol use.

How should you respond to his dyslipidemia?

    A. Start a low-dose statin despite elevated ALT.
    B. Further restrict his diet and recheck.
    C. Encourage more exercise and recheck.
    D. Recheck ALT every 6 months and start a statin once ALT is normal.
    E. Determine his LDL particle size.

285.

A new patient is seen in your clinic complaining of palpitations, tremors, heat intolerance, weight loss, hair loss, three bowel movements every day, and fatigue. He has a mild goiter that is nontender, smooth, symmetrical, and without nodules. There is no cervical lymphadenopathy. Feeling confident about diagnosing Graves disease, you prescribe a β-blocker for his symptoms and order TSH, FT4, and a thyroid scan and uptake. He returns in 2 weeks. His symptoms are much improved since taking the β-blocker, but he is still clinically hyperthyroid. The TSH is < 0.01 mU/L (0.5–5.0 mU/L) and FT4 is 2.5 ng/dL (0.7–1.5 ng/dL). The thyroid scan reveals a symmetrical goiter that is homogeneous. The thyroid uptake is 30% (10–35%).

What is most likely to explain his normal uptake?

    A. Hashimoto's thyroiditis
    B. Use of expired radioactive iodine by the nuclear medicine technician
    C. Low dietary intake of iodine
    D. High dietary intake of iodine
    E. Presence of multiple hot nodules

286.

55-year-old woman comes to your clinic for a routine visit. She has rheumatoid arthritis. Her rheumatologist has been treating her for the last 2 months with 5 mg of prednisone daily and intends to continue this therapy for the foreseeable future. She has a history of esophageal stricture. She gets limited exercise and avoids sun exposure as much as possible because it worsens her skin manifestations.

To lower her risk of developing glucocorticoid-induced osteoporosis, which of the following do you recommend?

    A. Encourage weight-bearing exercises.
    B. Continue to discourage sun exposure because of risk of melanoma.
    C. Begin calcium 4 g per day.
    D. Begin vitamin D 100 units per day.
    E. Begin an oral bisphosphonate.

287.

A mother brings her 18-year-old son to see you because his science teacher thinks something may be wrong. The class was learning to identify Barr bodies on buccal smears when it was noticed that the young man was the only male in the class with a Barr body. His mother says that he is timid and doesn't do well in school. Lately, the other boys have been making fun of him. His mother reports that he had the mumps at age 16. After his mother leaves the room, you ask him about erections and masturbation. He denies them both. You examine him and find that his arm span is 70 inches and his height is 69 inches. His testes are very small (< 1 in) and quite firm. He has mild bilateral gynecomastia and sparse facial hair. He reports that he hasn't started shaving yet. You order labs and have him come back to see you in 2 weeks. The following are the laboratory tests:

Chem-7 WNL
CBC WNL
Testosterone low for age and gender
FSH high for age and gender
LH high for age and gender

Which of the following do you tell him?

    A. He has Klinefelter syndrome and should start testosterone, 100 mg IM weekly.
    B. He has Kallmann syndrome and should start testosterone, 100 mg IM weekly.
    C. He suffers from primary hypogonadism due to post-pubertal mumps infection.
    D. He has hypogonadotropic hypogonadism.
    E. He has complete testicular feminization.

288.

You are asked to consult on a patient who was admitted to the medicine service with a severe headache followed by unconsciousness. He was found to have a history of a moderate-sized null cell tumor and apparently experienced apoplexy. The neurosurgeon relieved the pressure within the sella but reported extensive damage to the pituitary. The internist taking care of the patient tells you about the development of diabetes insipidus that lasted about 5 days, but the patient suddenly developed SIADH two days ago.

Which of the following best describes your appropriate response?

A. Begin dexamethasone and order a CRH-stimulation test to assess ACTH secretion.
B. Order a TSH test and begin thyroxine while waiting for the results.
C. Tell the other internist that the patient will probably soon go back into diabetes insipidus, which will most likely be permanent and require desmopressin (DDAVP®).
D. Follow the patient's volume status, urine, and serum sodium carefully.
E. All of the choices are correct.

289.

A young man comes to your office complaining about breast development. He denies taking any medications or illicit drugs. He has never used marijuana and doesn't even drink. His beard has gotten heavier, and he now has to shave twice a day. The rest of his history is negative, and your physical examination shows only mild bilateral gynecomastia and normal-sized but soft testes. You order some hormone tests and learn that his testosterone, estradiol, and dehydroepiandrosterone (DHEA) levels are elevated and his gonadotropins (LH and FSH) are low.

What do you suspect?

A. He is taking exogenous testosterone though he denies it.
B. He is taking exogenous estrogens though he denies it.
C. He has Klinefelter syndrome.
D. He has a testicular tumor secreting testosterone.
E. He has an adrenal tumor secreting dehydroepiandrosterone.

290.

A woman comes to your clinic complaining of weight gain and depression. On physical examination, you find moon facies, cervicodorsal fat pad (buffalo hump), central obesity, plethora, and some bruises. She tells you that she is depressed. You suspect Cushing syndrome and begin the workup.

Which of the following is true?

A. An elevated 24-hour urine cortisol diagnoses Cushing disease.
B. A low-dose overnight suppression test uses 0.5 mg of dexamethasone.
C. A normal 24-hour urine cortisol (10–90 µg/day) essentially excludes Cushing syndrome.
D. A low-dose overnight suppression test uses 2 mg of dexamethasone.
E. An overnight dexamethasone suppression test essentially excludes Cushing's syndrome if the morning cortisol is 6–10 µg/dL.

291.

An elderly man comes to your clinic at the insistence of his children. Ever since his wife died last year, he has been depressed and losing weight. He moved closer to his children after her death. He smokes 2 packs a day, having started smoking in 1942 while in the army. He is taking propranolol prescribed by his physician in his previous hometown, who was apparently treating him for mild hypertension. He talks to you easily, but doesn't seem very interested. His heart rate is 89, blood pressure 128/80, height 5'10", weight 160 lbs., and BMI 23.0 kg/m². The physical examination is unremarkable. You order a routine metabolic profile and CBC. You also order a chest x-ray because of his extensive smoking history. He comes back for the results in two weeks, and you tell him that the labs and x-ray were normal.

Which of the following would you do next?

A. Begin low-dose fluoxetine for his depression.
B. Order a CT scan of the chest.
C. Order a total body CT scan.
D. Check TSH and FT4.
E. Discontinue his propranolol and begin treating his hypertension with a thiazide diuretic.

292.

A 65-year-old woman is evaluated after sustaining a fractured wrist. She underwent menopause at age 48 and never took estrogen replacement therapy. She has a history of mild hypertension controlled with HCTZ 25 mg/day. She does not smoke and takes no other medications except calcium carbonate 500 mg daily. Bone mineral density testing shows a T score of –2.7 lumbar spine and –3.1 femoral neck.

Laboratory:
Serum calcium	11.1 (8.6–10.4 mg/dL)
Serum phosphorus	3.1 (2.5–4.5 mg/dL)
iPTH	49 (10–65 pg/mL)
TSH	0.5 (0.5–5.5 mU/L)
25(OH)-vitamin D	25.6 (20–100 ng/mL)

Which of the following should be the next step in this patient's management?

A. Check Free T4 level.
B. Stop HCTZ and calcium tablets and repeat serum calcium in 4 weeks.
C. Refer the patient for parathyroid surgery.
D. Treat the patient with vitamin D for 8 weeks and retest serum calcium and PTH.
E. Begin alendronate therapy.

293.

A 41-year-old woman is evaluated in the Emergency Department for headaches, which have been worsening over the past 6 months. She takes no medications and has no past medical history. She denies fatigue or facial flushing. She has not lost weight but has noted palpitations. She has no family history of hypertension. BP is 188/106 supine and 156/92 after standing. HR is 100 without change. Her thyroid is of normal size, cardiac exam is normal, and she has no pedal edema.

Laboratory:
Serum sodium	135 mEq/L (135–145 mEq/L)
Serum potassium	3.9 mEq/L (3.5–5.3 mEq/L)
Serum glucose (fasting)	139 mg/dL (80–126 mg/dL)

Which step is best for her subsequent management?

A. Measure serum aldosterone and plasma renin activity.
B. Measure serum cortisol at 8 a.m. after 1 mg dexamethasone at midnight.
C. Perform CT of the abdomen with IV contrast.
D. Measure plasma fractionated catecholamines.
E. Measure 24-hour urine fractionated metanephrines.

294.

An elderly woman comes to your clinic complaining of weakness, fatigue, and having no interest in life. On questioning, she reports cold intolerance, one bowel movement every 4–5 days, and some hair loss but denies any weight gain. She is depressed and doesn't care about herself or her home. BP 98/62 and HR 57.

Laboratory:
Na^+	140 mEq/L (135–143 mEq/L)
K^+	4.9 mEq/L (3.5–5.0 mEq/L)
Cl^-	109 mEq/L (100–109 mEq/L)
HCO_3^-	21 mEq/L (22–30 mEq/L)
Urea nitrogen	9 mg/dL (8–18 mg/dL)
Creatinine	0.9 mg/dL (0.6–1.2 mg/dL)
Glucose	72 mg/dL (65–110 mg/dL)
FT4	0.3 ng/dL (0.7–1.5 ng/dL)
TSH	14.6 mU/L (0.5–5.0 mU/L).

Which of the following should you do now?

A. Begin oral thyroxine 300 μg qd.
B. Begin oral thyroxine 50 μg qd.
C. Begin oral thyroxine 100 μg qd.
D. Begin oral dexamethasone 0.5 mg q a.m. first, and then oral thyroxine 100 μg per day, and perform an $ACTH_{1-24}$ (cosyntropin) stimulation test.
E. Give one dose of IV thyroxine 500 μg in "one-day stay" and begin oral thyroxine 150 μg qd.

295.

You are asked to see an elderly woman with CHF in the CCU. The cardiologist tells you that the patient just isn't responding to treatment like she should. You find her somnolent but easy to arouse and in good spirits. She reports recent fatigue and edema at the nursing home. Your examination reveals normal body hair but dry skin. She has lower extremity and periorbital edema. Heart rate is 64 with a third heart sound. The lungs have bilateral anterolateral crackles. A recent echo showed some left ventricular wall abnormalities and a mildly decreased ejection fraction, but no pericardial effusion. You order thyroid tests, which come back as the following:

FT4   0.3 ng/dL (0.7–1.5 ng/dL)
TSH   58 mU/L (0.5–5.0 mU/L).

What is your recommendation at this time?

A. Check reverse T3 (rT3) for suspected euthyroid sick syndrome.
B. Begin intravenous thyroxine therapy for rapid return to normal.
C. Begin intravenous thyroxine and triiodothyronine (T3) to replace the missing T3 and to saturate the unused binding sites of thyroxine binding globulin.
D. Oral thyroxine 200 μg per day and oral triiodothyronine (T3) 25 μg per day.
E. Begin oral thyroxine 12.5 μg per day while closely watching her cardiac status.

296.

You are covering for a colleague one week when a diabetic comes to see you for her routine visit. She is 53 years old, has a history of diabetic neuropathy, and has an early foot ulcer. She checks her glucose and reports that her morning glucose is generally 90–120. She takes metformin 500 mg twice daily and a baby aspirin every day. She also has been taking cephalexin, prescribed by an Infectious Disease expert who is following the foot ulcer closely. She doesn't smoke and her blood pressure is 130/78. Her recent lab results are as follows and are not much different from her last visit:

Na^+	140 mEq/L (135–143 mEq/L)
K^+	4.2 mEq/L (3.5–5.0 mEq/L)
Cl^-	104 mEq/L (100–109 mEq/L)
HCO_3^-	24 mEq/L (22–30 mEq/L)
Urea nitrogen	15 mg/dL (8–18 mg/dL)
Creatinine	1.4 mg/dL (0.6–1.2 mg/dL)
Glucose	143 mg/dL (65–110 mg/dL)
Total bilirubin	0.3 mg/dL (0.1–1.0 mg/dL)
HbA1c	8.1 % (4.9–6.2 %)
LDL	140 mg/dL
HDL	34 mg/dL
TG	179 mg/dL
WBC	$9.8 \times 10^3/\mu L$ (4.5–$11.0 \times 10^3/\mu L$).

Which of the following is the most important action for you to take at this time?

   A. Add an additional oral agent.
   B. Increase the metformin to 1,000 mg twice daily.
   C. Stop the metformin and start a different oral agent.
   D. Add an antibiotic that offers *Pseudomonas* coverage.
   E. Begin a statin.

297.

A 28-year-old woman is evaluated for a 6-month history of amenorrhea. Prior to cessation of cycles, she was experiencing heavy bleeding. She had an uneventful labor and delivery 2 years earlier. She takes fluoxetine 40 mg daily. There is a family history of maternal Graves disease. She complains of some fatigue and occasional headaches. On physical exam, BP is 130/90 and clear fluid is expressible from her nipples. MRI of the sella is obtained and reveals a homogenous mass measuring 1.3 cm in height.

Laboratory:

Basal metabolic panel		Normal
LH	3.1 mIU/mL	(1.9–12.5 mIU/mL)
FSH	2.2 mIU/mL	(2.5–10.2 mIU/mL)
Estradiol	41 pg/mL	(30–375 pg/mL)
Prolactin	106 ng/mL	(3–28 ng/mL)

Which of the following is the next step in her management?

A. Check serum 17-OH-progesterone level.
B. Check a visual field examination.
C. Check serum TSH.
D. Begin therapy with cabergoline 0.5 mg twice weekly.
E. Refer the patient for neurosurgical consultation.

298.

A 25-year-old woman comes to see you for irregular menses and difficulty getting pregnant. She denies unusual stress or any recent changes in her health. Her periods were regular until 8 months ago. She briskly walks 1 mile 4 days per week and has been dieting for 1 year. Her weight has decreased 47 pounds during the previous year. Your physical examination shows a small thyroid nodule and somewhat brisk deep tendon reflexes.

You order a series of tests and have her return in 3 weeks to discuss the results, which are as follows:

Na^+	140 mEq/L (135–143 mEq/L)
K^+	4.0 mEq/L (3.5–5.0 mEq/L)
Cl^-	104 mEq/L (100–109 mEq/L)
HCO_3^-	24 mEq/L (22–30 mEq/L)
Urea nitrogen	9 mg/dL (8–18 mg/dL)
Creatinine	0.8 mg/dL (0.6–1.2 mg/dL)
Glucose	85 mg/dL (65–110 mg/dL)
Ca^{+2}	9.9 mg/dL (8.5–10.5 mg/dL)
FT4	1.9 ng/dL (0.7–1.5 ng/dL)
TSH	0.01 mU/L (0.5–5.0 mU/L).

Pelvic ultrasound was normal.
Nuclear medicine thyroid scan showed mildly enlarged thyroid with generally diffuse uptake, except for a 1.5 cm cold nodule.
Nuclear medicine thyroid uptake was 40% (normal 10–35%).

Which of the following recommendations should be given to her at this time?

A. PTU 100 mg every 8 hours with follow-up in 2 months.
B. Surgical resection of her thyroid, followed by thyroxine replacement.
C. Ultrasound-guided biopsy of her thyroid nodule.
D. Radioactive iodine ablation of the thyroid gland, avoid getting pregnant for at least 6 months, and biopsy the nodule if it still exists after the ablation.
E. Begin oral contraceptives and repeat the thyroid tests in 6 months.

299.

A new elderly patient comes to your clinic in Philadelphia one winter day complaining about fatigue. His past medical history is insignificant. On examination, you find him to be thin and well tanned, but with sparse pubic hair and no axillary hair. BP 96/62 and HR 109. Chem-7 shows the following:

Na^+	138 mEq/L (135–143 mEq/L)
K^+	5.3 mEq/L (3.5–5.0 mEq/L)

Cl⁻	108 mEq/L (100–109 mEq/L)
HCO_3^-	19 mEq/L (22–30 mEq/L)
Urea nitrogen	9 mg/dL (8–18 mg/dL)
Creatinine	0.9 mg/dL (0.6–1.2 mg/dL)
Glucose	66 mg/dL (65–110 mg/dL).

At this point, you make an initial diagnosis and plan the appropriate workup.

Which of the following is the initial diagnosis?

    A. Pseudo adrenal insufficiency
    B. Secondary adrenal insufficiency
    C. Primary adrenal insufficiency
    D. Hypothyroidism
    E. Glucocorticoid abuse

300.

A patient recently passed a kidney stone in the local Emergency Department and is referred to your clinic for follow-up. He is a "health freak" and takes megadoses of vitamins and supplements of calcium. As part of your workup, you obtain the following labs:

Na⁺	140 mEq/L (135–143 mEq/L)
K⁺	4.0 mEq/L (3.5–5.0 mEq/L)
Cl⁻	104 mEq/L (100–109 mEq/L)
HCO_3^-	24 mEq/L (22–30 mEq/L)
Urea nitrogen	12 mg/dL (8–18 mg/dL)
Creatinine	1.6 mg/dL (0.6–1.2 mg/dL)
Glucose	85 mg/dL (65–110 mg/dL)
Ca^{+2}	10.6 mg/dL (8.5–10.5 mg/dL)
Phosphate	2.5 mg/dL (2.5–4.5 mg/dL)
Albumin	4.6 g/dL (4.0–6.0 g/dL)
Vitamin A	120 µg/dL (30–100 µg/dL)

25OH-Vitamin D	80 µg/L (10–55 µg/L)
1,25(OH)₂-Vit D	68 ng/L (18–62 ng/L)
intact PTH	42 pg/mL (10–65 pg/mL).

Which of the following is the most likely cause of his hypercalcemia?

    A. Unknown malignancy
    B. Primary hyperparathyroidism
    C. Granulomatous disease
    D. Vitamin A toxicosis
    E. Vitamin D toxicosis

301.

A 25-year-old woman presents with a 3-week history of palpitations, anxiety, fatigue, and difficulty sleeping. She notes a 5-pound weight loss. She denies recent viral infections, fever, or change in her vision. Her mother is receiving thyroid replacement. On examination, BP 110/76, pulse 104, the thyroid gland is enlarged twice normal on the right and three times normal on the left and is not tender. There is no exophthalmos.

Laboratory:
CBC   normal
ESR   31
TSH   < 0.01 mIU/L (0.5–5.0 mIU/L)
Free T4   2.8 ng/dL   (0.7–1.6 ng/dL)

Which of these possible next steps would be most helpful in her subsequent management?

A. Measure 24-hour thyroid uptake of ^{131}I.
B. Perform thyroid ultrasound.
C. Measure anti-thyroid peroxidase antibodies.
D. Measure serum free T3 level.
E. Begin therapy with methimazole.

302.

Which of the following thyroid disorders will cause a high nuclear medicine thyroid uptake?

A. Postpartum thyroiditis
B. Amiodarone
C. Graves disease
D. Iodine excess
E. Subacute thyroiditis

303.

A 49-year-old man presents for a follow-up exam. He was diagnosed with Type 2 diabetes 10 years ago. Current therapy includes metformin 500 mg bid and glyburide 5 mg bid. He is also treated for hypertension with hydrochlorothiazide 25 mg/day. He does not test blood glucose at home. He feels well. BMI = 44; BP is 145/90; he has no edema. Funduscopic exam is unremarkable.

Laboratory:
Serum creatinine   0.8 mg/dL (0.5–1.4 mg/dL)
Hemoglobin A1c   8.8% (4–6%)
Fasting plasma triglycerides   1,077 (< 150 mg/dL)
Urine microalbumin-creatinine ratio 131 (0–30 mcg/mg)

Which of the following is the best set of adjustments for his therapeutic regimen?

 A. Increase metformin to 1,000 mg bid, increase glyburide to 10 mg bid, and begin gemfibrozil.
 B. Increase glyburide to 10 mg bid, begin lisinopril, and begin pravastatin.
 C. Begin enalapril, begin fenofibrate, and begin insulin glargine.
 D. Begin 70/30 insulin bid, stop metformin, and increase HCTZ to 50 mg/day.
 E. Stop glyburide, begin 70/30 insulin bid, begin amlodipine 5 mg/day.

304.

A thin, elderly man slipped in his bathtub and was knocked unconscious. His wife called the ambulance. He recovered before the ambulance got him to the hospital. A CT scan of his head was normal, except for a 2 mm pituitary mass. The physician in the Emergency Department referred him to you for follow-up. Your examination shows nothing to be out of the ordinary except for numerous skin tags and a fasting glucose of 128 mg/dL. He had a screening colonoscopy 8 months ago that found several small polyps that were all benign. A 24-hour Holter monitor failed to show any arrhythmias.

Which of the following is the most appropriate next step?

 A. Repeat the head CT in 6 months.
 B. Check a 24-hour urine cortisol to exclude Cushing disease.
 C. Refer him to a neurosurgeon for possible resection of the mass.
 D. Check the IGF-1 level because you suspect acromegaly.
 E. Recheck the fasting glucose next month for possible diabetes.

305.

A 56-year-old woman comes to see you for a routine Pap smear and general checkup. She reports mild fatigue but continues with a very active lifestyle, including tennis one day a week and a 2-mile brisk walk 5 days per week. Her past medical history is unremarkable, she doesn't smoke, and she is taking over-the-counter calcium supplements. The physical exam is unremarkable, and the Pap smear is done without difficulty. You tell her that she will probably dance on your grave. You order some blood tests and tell her to call for the results next week. The Pap smear is normal.

Laboratory:
Na^+	140 mEq/L (135–143 mEq/L)
K^+	4.0 mEq/L (3.5–5.0 mEq/L)
Cl^-	104 mEq/L (100–109 mEq/L)
HCO_3^-	24 mEq/L (22–30 mEq/L)
Urea nitrogen	9 mg/dL (8–18 mg/dL)
Creatinine	0.8 mg/dL (0.6–1.2 mg/dL)
Glucose	92 mg/dL (65–110 mg/dL)
Ca^{+2}	9.7 mg/dL (8.5–10.5 mg/dL)
FT4	0.9 ng/dL (0.7–1.5 ng/dL)
TSH	4.6 mU/L (0.5–5.0 mU/L)

Fasting lipids:
LDL	195 mg/dL
HDL	41 mg/dL
TG	107 mg/dL.

Which of the following is the best plan of action at this time?

A. Recommend a diet low in cholesterol and saturated fat.
B. Begin thyroxine 50 μg per day and check lipids, TSH, FT4, and anti-thyroid antibodies in 2–3 months.
C. Order a 75-gram oral glucose tolerance test (OGTT) to rule out diabetes.
D. Schedule a revisit appointment in one year.
E. Order a baseline bone density study to rule out osteoporosis.

306.

An elderly man with benign prostatic hyperplasia (BPH) is scheduled for a TURP. He has complete obstruction and required a suprapubic catheter. He now has post-obstruction diuresis and a concentrating defect. The surgeon is having difficulty managing the patient's fluid status and electrolytes. He wants to perform the TURP as soon as possible and has consulted you for medical clearance. During your examination, you find a small goiter, tachycardia, and A-fib as well as prostatic hypertrophy, a suprapubic catheter, and a large volume of dilute urine, but the urine osmolality is improving. Because of the tachyarrhythmia, you check his thyroid function. The lab reports TSH < 0.01 mU/L (normal 0.5–5.0 mU/L) and FT4 2.4 ng/dL (normal 0.7–1.5 ng/dL). The patient does not have anyone at home to help him and cannot go home with a suprapubic catheter. He has no insurance and cannot afford home health care.

Your consult includes multiple recommendations, but which of the following is <u>not</u> included?

A. Begin PTU 200 μg every 8 hours.
B. Begin a β-blocker.
C. Begin anticoagulants.
D. Avoid contrast dye and anything else that contains iodine so he can be referred for radioactive iodine ablation after surgery.
E. Postpone surgery until his FT4 is within normal limits.

307.

A 40-year-old man presents with several unique complaints. He has noted for some time that his voice was deepening and that he seems to sweat a lot. He went skiing last week, and, when he placed his helmet on his head, he noted that it no longer fit properly—the helmet seemed to be too small.

On physical examination you note frontal bossing and coarse facial features.

Thinking you know the diagnosis, which test would help you confirm it?

A. Random growth hormone level; should be > 5 ng/mL in this patient.
B. Growth hormone level 1 hour and 2 hours after 100-gram glucose load; this should be > 5 ng/mL in this patient.
C. Growth hormone level 1 hour and 2 hours after 100-gram glucose load; this should be < 5 ng/mL in this patient.
D. Simultaneous glucose and growth hormone levels at bedtime and 4 a.m.; look for a 3-fold rise in growth hormone.
E. Growth hormone levels after a 12-hour fast; look for growth hormone > 5 ng/mL.

308.

Jessica Simpleton is a 40-year-old woman who presents with proximal muscle weakness and depression. Your physician assistant saw her initially and ordered a series of tests after examining her last week.

Physical Exam: BP 150/100, P 110, RR 20, Temp 99° F
      HEENT: Moon facies, acne
      Hirsutism
      Heart: RRR with I/VI systolic murmur
      Lungs: CTA
      Abdomen: Central obesity, prominent striae
      Extremities: Thin arms and legs
      Buffalo hump
      Supraclavicular fat pads noted

Laboratory:
24-hour urine cortisol: 250 µg/day (normal 20–90 µg/day)
1-mg dexamethasone test: morning cortisol level after p.m. dose given: 18 µg/dL (normal < 5 µg/dL)
8-mg dexamethasone test: morning cortisol level after p.m. dose given: < 50% of baseline cortisol level

What is the most likely etiology for her symptoms?

    A. Hypothyroidism
    B. Cushing disease
    C. Ectopic ACTH production
    D. Pseudo-Cushing syndrome
    E. High stress levels

309.

A 16-year-old high school student is referred for evaluation of amenorrhea. She is an "A" student and has been active in school activities. She denies any other health problems.

Physical Examination:
      Vital signs BP 140/80, P 60, RR 18, Temp 98.7° F
      Height 4' 4"; weight 130 lbs
      HEENT: Wears glasses; otherwise normal
      Neck: Possible short neck
      Heart: RRR with II-III/VI systolic murmur
      Lungs: CTA
      Breast: Tanner Stage I-II; widely spaced nipples
      Abdomen: +BS, soft, No Hepatosplenomegaly
      Extremities: Short legs noted
      GU: Normal pubic hair distribution

Based on your findings, what do you expect her LH, FSH levels to be?

    A. Her LH will be low, FSH high.
    B. Her LH will be high, FSH high.
    C. Her LH will be low, FSH low.
    D. Her LH will be high, FSH low.
    E. It depends on what time of day you draw the levels.

310.

A 25-year-old man presents because he and his wife have been unable to conceive. He denies any medical problems and has been healthy most of his life.

Past Medical History: Negative

Social History: Works as a ski instructor in the winter; Works as a tennis instructor in the summer

Family History: Unknown, was adopted

Review of Systems: Has noted that his sense of smell doesn't seem to be as good as that of other people's. His wife gets upset with him because he doesn't notice her perfume.

Physical Examination: 6'4" tall, weight 180 lbs.
Body Habitus: Eunuchoid proportioned—His lower body segment > upper body segment. His arm span is 7 cm more than his height.
GU exam: Testes are small for age, only 3 cm

Which of the following is true with regard to his diagnosis?

    A. A karyotype will be diagnostic.
    B. His basal FSH and LH levels will be low or undetectable.
    C. Testosterone levels will be undetectable.
    D. His mental development is abnormally high for this diagnosis.
    E. If GnRH is given, FSH and LH will respond appropriately.

311.

A 27-year-old woman presents with complaints of easy fatigability and recent occurrence of milky discharge from her nipples. She is the mother of an 11-month-old girl but has not nursed in 6 months. She has not started to menstruate since the pregnancy. The discharge began about 6 weeks ago. She denies headaches or visual disturbances. She is on no medications currently. Physical examination is normal except for the presence of galactorrhea. Her prolactin level is 208 ng/mL (elevated).

Which of the following statements is true?

    A. Empty-sella syndrome needs to be investigated.
    B. Hypothyroidism is likely.
    C. Pregnancy must be ruled out.
    D. Most likely she has a prolactinoma.
    E. This is a common, benign, post-pregnancy condition.

312.

A 35-year-old man presents for a pre-work physical. He is normal, except that you note he has extremely small testicles and prominent gynecomastia. He says that no one else in his family has a similar body type to himself.

Laboratory:
GnRH: High
FSH: High
LH: High
Ferritin: Normal
Prolactin level: Normal

What is his karyotype?

    A. XX
    B. XY
    C. XYY
    D. XXY
    E. XXXXXXXXy

313.

A 21-year-old man comes in for evaluation of polyuria and polydipsia.

Here are his initial laboratory values:
Serum sodium   144 mg/dL
Serum potassium   4 mg/dL
Serum chloride   107 mg/dL
Serum bicarbonate   25 mg/dL
BUN   18 mg/dL
Glucose   102 mg/dL
Urine sodium   28 mg/dL
Urine potassium   32 mg/dL
Urine osmolality: 195 mosmol/kg water

Okay … You fluid-deprive him for 12 hours and his body weight falls 5%!!

Now, now you send for laboratory again:
Serum sodium: 150 mg/dL
Serum potassium   4 mg/dL
Serum chloride   110 mg/dL
Serum bicarbonate   25 mg/dL
BUN   19 mg/dL
Glucose   100 mg/dL
Urine sodium   24 mg/dL
Urine potassium   35 mg/dL
Urine osmolality: 200 mosmol/kg water

Now, you give him 5 units of arginine vasopressin subcutaneously, and his urine values 1 hour later show:

Urine sodium	30 mg/dL
Urine potassium	30 mg/dL
Urine osmolality	199 mosmol/kg water

Given these lab results, which of the following is his most likely diagnosis?

    A. Osmotic diuresis
    B. Salt-losing nephropathy
    C. Psychogenic polydipsia
    D. Nephrogenic diabetes insipidus
    E. Lupus nephritis

314.

A 22-year-old woman presents with weight loss and fatigue. She had an episode of near syncope which brought her to seek medical attention. Her last menstrual cycle was 4 months ago. She complains of abdominal pain, nausea, and anorexia. Her older sister has Type 1 diabetes and primary hypothyroidism. Supine BP is 100/60, HR 92, but standing BP is 66/40. Abdomen is soft and nontender. Urine β-HCG is negative.

Laboratory studies:
Urinalysis is unremarkable.
Serum sodium is 128 mEq/L

Which of the following is most likely to lead to the correct diagnosis?

    A. Measure plasma glucose.
    B. Measure serum potassium.
    C. Measure free T4 and TSH.
    D. Measure serum cortisol before and after cosyntropin (Cortrosyn™) injection.
    E. Measure HbA1c.

HEMATOLOGY

315.

A patient presents with mental status changes and confusion. A CBC is available, and the platelet count is 5,000.

The appropriate workup should include which of the following?

A. An LDH, bilirubin, and chemistries.
B. A reticulocyte count.
C. A review of the peripheral smear.
D. All of the choices are correct.
E. None of the choices are correct.

316.

A young woman presents with new onset of a DVT. She has a history of spontaneous fetal loss 2 years prior but no acute problems. Her lab studies include a baseline PT and aPTT. Her PT is normal but her aPTT is prolonged 5 secs.

An appropriate evaluation would include which of the following?

A. Mixing studies.
B. Lupus anticoagulant.
C. Antiphospholipid antibody screening.
D. All of the choices are correct.
E. None of choices are correct.

317.

A 76-year-old man presents with enlarging adenopathy in his cervical region. He has no other symptoms and otherwise feels well. He has a biopsy and the pathology report shows a low-grade lymphoma (small lymphocytic lymphoma).

Appropriate evaluation and treatment should include all of the following except:

A. Bone marrow aspirate and biopsy
B. CT scans of chest, abdomen, and pelvis
C. High-dose chemotherapy followed by bone marrow transplant
D. Observation

318.

A patient is referred from the Emergency Department for evaluation of anemia. Her hemoglobin and hematocrit are mildly depressed (10 and 30, respectively), and her MCV is 62. Her peripheral smear is noted to have many target cells.

The most appropriate evaluation should include which of the following?

A. Iron, iron-binding capacity, ferritin.
B. Hemoglobin electrophoresis.
C. Reticulocyte count.
D. All of the choices are correct.
E. None of the choices are correct.

319.

You are asked to see a patient who complains of easy bruising. She describes bleeding gums and bruising for 2–3 weeks. A CBC has a WBC of 55,000 with many immature forms. Her PT and PTT are prolonged. A bone marrow confirms your diagnosis of acute leukemia, and the Sudan stain is positive. She appears to be in DIC.

Which of the following subtypes of AML does this patient likely have?

A. M0
B. M3
C. M6
D. M7
E. M9

320.

A 90-year-old is referred for pancytopenia. His peripheral smear shows a microcytic anemia and WBCs that are described as pseudo-Pelger-Huët forms.

Which of the following statements is true?

A. His bone marrow is likely to be aplastic.
B. His bone marrow is likely to be hypercellular with dysplasia in all cell lines.
C. He has acute leukemia.
D. He has essential thrombocytosis.
E. He has a curable illness.

321.

A patient presents with a platelet count of over 1 million discovered on routine CBC. She is asymptomatic. She denies any bleeding or symptoms suggestive of stroke.

The most common etiology for her problem is which of the following?

A. Acute leukemia
B. Essential thrombocytosis
C. Iron deficiency
D. Occult malignancy
E. High altitude

322.

A 65-year-old man presents with complaints of pain in his hip. He has an x-ray, which identifies a single lytic lesion.

Which of the following should be done next?

A. A bone marrow aspirate and biopsy
B. A bone scan
C. A serum protein electrophoresis and urine electrophoresis
D. A β-HCG and alpha-fetoprotein
E. Observation with repeat x-rays in 6 weeks

323.

An elderly patient presents with pneumonia and is noted by CBC to have a WBC count of 90,000 with mostly lymphocytes. Some of the lymphocytes are atypical. The hemoglobin and platelet counts are normal.

Which of the following is the most likely diagnosis?

A. An acute viral illness
B. A leukemoid reaction
C. Chronic myeloid leukemia
D. Chronic lymphocytic leukemia

324.

A patient presents with a RBC count that is elevated, with a hemoglobin of 17 g/dL, and a hematocrit of 52%. The WBC count is also elevated (19,000), and the platelet count is 550,000. The patient describes early satiety and by exam has splenomegaly.

Appropriate diagnostic studies could include which of the following?

A. A RBC mass.
B. An erythropoietin level.
C. A bone marrow for cytogenetics.
D. An oxygen saturation test.
E. All of the choices are correct.

325.

A 50-year-old man presents with complaints of early satiety, weight loss, and fatigue. He denies any recent infectious complications. His physical exam is pertinent for splenomegaly.

Which of the following is <u>not</u> likely?

A. Chronic myeloid leukemia (CML)
B. Chronic lymphocytic leukemia (CLL)
C. Hairy cell leukemia
D. Aplastic anemia
E. Non-Hodgkin lymphoma

326.

A 40-year-old woman presents with fatigue, epistaxis, and complaints of a rash on her lower extremities. Her family has noticed some confusion over the last 1–2 days. Her physical exam is pertinent only for pallor and petechia on her legs.

Laboratory:

Hemoglobin	7 g/dL
Hematocrit	21%
WBC count	150,000/μL
Platelet count	22,000/μL

The differential for the WBC count is:

Segmented neutrophils	5%
Monocytes	5%
Lymphocytes	10%
Blasts	80%

Which of the following statements is true?

A. A blast count of > 100,000 never requires intervention.
B. Auer rods in the blasts would indicate an acute myeloid leukemia.
C. Cytogenetics are unimportant for prognosis in this illness.
D. M4 and M5 subtypes of acute myeloid leukemia are typically associated with DIC.
E. Radiation therapy is the treatment of choice for this disorder.

327.

A 50-year-old woman is seen and diagnosed with breast cancer. She receives chemotherapy, including the drug mitomycin C. She presents 3 days later with fever and confusion. Her CBC is as follows:

	Pretreatment:	Current:
Hemoglobin	13 g/dL	6 g/dL
Hematocrit	39%	18%
WBC count	5,000/μL	4,800/μL
Platelet count	283,000/μL	22,000/μL

The most appropriate next step would include which of the following?

A. Order LDH, total and fractionated bilirubin, reticulocyte count, review peripheral smear; proceed with emergent therapeutic plasma exchange.
B. Blood cultures and antibiotic therapy.
C. Immediate platelet transfusion.
D. Admit for observation and repeat CBC in the morning.
E. Treatment with growth factors such as erythropoietin and G-CSF.

328.

A 25-year-old woman presents with a new occlusive lower-extremity DVT. She denies any trauma or prolonged immobilization. She is currently on no medications other than an occasional aspirin product. Routine workup reveals:

Left leg Doppler positive for an acute occlusive thrombosis
Hematocrit   39%
WBC count   6,000/µL
Platelet count 393,000/µL
PT   12.1 sec (control of 11.9)
aPTT   50 sec (control of 36)

Appropriate evaluation and intervention includes all of the following <u>except</u>:

A. Mix patient's plasma 1:1 with normal plasma to assess for correction of the aPTT.
B. Do not acutely treat patient with anticoagulation since she is already anticoagulated (aPTT prolonged).
C. Treat with low-molecular weight heparin (LMWH) and then add warfarin for a target INR of 2–3.
D. ANA screen.
E. Tentative diagnosis is antiphospholipid antibody syndrome (APLA).

329.

A 70-year-old man presents with complaints of neck swelling and early satiety. He denies any recent infections or exposures. By physical exam, he has multiple 2–3 cm lymph nodes in the cervical chains and supraclavicular areas on both sides. He has a spleen tip palpable with deep inspiration.

His laboratory results are pertinent for a CBC with the following results:
Hemoglobin   9 g/dL
Hematocrit   27%
WBC count   60,000/µL
Platelet count 103,333/µL

The differential for the WBC count is:
        20% Segmented neutrophils
        5% Prolymphocytes
        75% Lymphocytes

Which of the following statements is correct about this syndrome?

    A. This is an aggressive illness and should be treated for cure.
    B. This disease is more common in younger patients.
    C. Autoimmune hemolytic anemia and ITP may be associated with this disease.
    D. This is stage I disease by the Rai staging system.
    E. Life expectancy with this is < 6 months.

330.

Which of the following has a prolonged PT, aPTT, and decreased fibrinogen?

    A. DIC.
    B. TTP.
    C. HIT.
    D. All of the choices are correct.
    E. None of the choices is correct.

331.

A 19-year-old patient with sickle cell disease is seen in your office for routine health maintenance. She has not had a crisis in over one year and currently takes only folate.

Her CBC has the following results:
Hemoglobin	6.5 g/dL
WBC count	20,000/μL
Hematocrit	18%
Platelet count	303,000/μL

Which of the following statements is true?

    A. She is not at higher risk for developing *Salmonella* osteomyelitis.
    B. She should be placed on hydroxyurea therapy.
    C. She should be started on a RBC exchange program to maintain an Hgb S level of < 40%.
    D. She is at risk for avascular necrosis, CVA, and aplastic crisis associated with parvovirus B19.
    E. She should be counseled to avoid pregnancy because all her offspring will be affected with sickle cell disease.

332.

A 63-year-old woman presents with complaints of progressive fatigue and dyspnea on exertion. She denies a history of cardiac or pulmonary disease. She has never been anemic and denies any bleeding. She had a total abdominal hysterectomy and bilateral salpingo-oophorectomy at age 46.

Her CBC today is as follows:
WBC count	4,500
Hemoglobin	8.4
Hematocrit	25.2%
Platelet count	752,000

MCV   75
RDW   20
Reticulocyte count: 2% (uncorrected)

Which of the following statements is true?

    A. Her lab results are diagnostic for essential thrombocytosis.
    B. She needs a hemoglobin electrophoresis for diagnosis.
    C. Her CBC is normal for her age.
    D. She should have a screening colonoscopy.
    E. No intervention is necessary at this time.

A 62-year-old man presents with complaints of fatigue, weight loss, and early satiety. His physical exam confirms a large spleen, but no lymphadenopathy is found.

His CBC is as follows:
Hematocrit   32%
WBC count   450,000
Platelet count 103,000

His differential is as follows:
Segmented neutrophils 30%,
Promyelocytes   5%
Bands   20%
Blasts   2%
Lymphocytes   10%,
Eosinophils   8%
Metamyelocytes   15%
Basophils   10%

You suspect a diagnosis of chronic myeloid leukemia.

Which of the following statements is true of CML?

    A. His prognosis is better if he is Philadelphia 1 chromosome [t(9,22)] negative.
    B. He should have a splenectomy for staging.
    C. During the natural course of this disease, more than 95% of patients develop acute myeloid leukemia.
    D. The Ph1+ chromosome [t(9,22)] produces an abnormal tyrosine kinase, which has been targeted by a new drug—imatinib (Gleevec®).
    E. The treatment of choice for this patient is immediate bone marrow transplant.

334.

A 35-year-old teacher is seen for pneumonia symptoms and found to have pancytopenia. Her physical exam is unremarkable except for a palpable spleen tip. The peripheral smear shows many lymphoid type cells, many of which have fine hair-like projections. You suspect hairy cell leukemia.

All of the following are true about hairy cell leukemia <u>except</u>:

A. Current treatment of choice is splenectomy.
B. The bone marrow is usually hypercellular with increased reticulin.
C. Diagnosis can be made with immuno-phenotyping.
D. The CD11c marker is relatively specific for hairy cell leukemia.
E. The bone is usually inaspirable (a dry tap).

335.

A 50-year-old male patient presents with primary complaints of fatigue and a lingering cold for one-month duration. He saw his regular physician last week and received a round of antibiotics; however, none of his symptoms improved. He was seen again yesterday and a CBC was drawn. He is unsure of the results but was told to come see you today for further evaluation. His past medical history is unremarkable except for hypertension. He takes hydrochlorothiazide 25 mg once daily. He works in a light bulb factory.

His physical exam reveals pallor and evidence of petechia. His heart has a 3/6 systolic ejection murmur throughout the precordium. His lungs are clear, and there is no organomegaly on abdominal exam.

No laboratory was sent with the patient so you request a CBC and chemistry panel. The results are as follows:

Hemoglobin	2.6
Hematocrit	10
WBC	500
Segs	15%
Lymphs	70%
Monos	10%
Eos	5%
Platelets	18,000
MCV	115
Na	135
K	4.0
Cl	112
HCO_3^-	23
BUN	26
Creat	1.2

Which of the following is the most appropriate next diagnostic step?

A. Lymphocyte subset typing (flow cytometry) to evaluate for CLL
B. A sternal bone marrow aspirate to evaluate for cellularity
C. Discontinuation of hydrochlorothiazide and follow-up in one week to assess a CBC again
D. A bone marrow aspirate and biopsy to assess for cellularity and the presence of infiltrative processes, such as acute leukemia
E. Check a B_{12} and folate level and empirically start B_{12} 1,000 mcg IM and folate 1 mg daily until the levels return

336.

A 45-year-old African-American female presents to your office on referral from the orthopedist. She originally saw him 4 weeks ago after falling and injuring her hip. She was found at that time to have a lytic lesion in her iliac crest, and a biopsy of that lesion was consistent with a plasmacytoma.

She has no previous medical history and has never had surgery. She does not smoke or drink alcohol. She takes no medications and has no drug allergies. There is no family history of malignancy.

Laboratory:

Hemoglobin	11
BUN	8
Hematocrit	35
Creatinine	0.9
Total protein	10
Calcium	9.5
Albumin	4.2
WBC	4,600
Segs	55%
Bands	3%
Lymphs	35%
Monos	7%
Platelets	450,000

SPE M-spike 2.3; IFE IgG Kappa monoclonal gammopathy.

She has had a bone marrow biopsy with < 10% plasma cells and otherwise normal results.

Appropriate management for this patient would include which of the following?

  A. Observation only since there is no indication for treatment. She should have serial SPEs and bone marrow exams every three months.
  B. Oral chemotherapy with agents such as melphalan and prednisone given every 4–6 weeks. Treatment should be given for only 6 cycles.
  C. Plans should be made for high-dose chemotherapy with peripheral blood stem cell rescue as front-line therapy.
  D. Radiation therapy to the lytic lesion followed by observation. Her M spike should be followed every 1–3 months for progression. She should be given a bisphosphonate for prevention of bony disease progression.

337.

A 36-year-old Caucasian female is admitted through the Emergency Department to your service. She complains of fatigue and a vague headache. She has not "felt well" for about a week but has progressively gotten weaker over the last 2 days. Last night, she noticed that she was unable to stand on her right leg and that there was no feeling in her foot. By the time she reached the hospital, these symptoms had all resolved.

She denies any previous medical history and has had no recent viral illnesses of which she is aware. She is on no chronic medications and has no drug allergies.

Her physical exam is really unremarkable, and there are no focal neurological deficits found. She does appear pale and has a soft flow murmur at the left upper sternal border.

Laboratory:

Hemoglobin 2.4	BUN 32	LDH 4,000	ALT 40
Hematocrit 10	Creatinine 2.2	T Protein 6.0	AST 52
WBC 8,900	SGGT 38	Albumin 4.0	

    Segs   89%
    Bands   2%
    Lymphs 9%

Platelets 3,000	Direct bilirubin 1.0	Total bilirubin 10.0

Reticulocyte count 12%

Prothrombin time 12 secs.
Activated partial thromboplastin time 39 secs
FDP 3
Fibrinogen 210

A CT scan of her head was normal.

Further workup and management should include which of the following?

    A. A bone marrow aspirate and biopsy to further investigate the cause of her cytopenia. She should receive a platelet transfusion prior to her procedure to prevent complications.

    B. Vitamin B_{12} and folate levels should be drawn and appropriate replacement given when the levels are available.

    C. Her peripheral smear should be reviewed for evidence of a microangiopathic picture. She should then be supported with replacement products such as fresh frozen plasma, cryoprecipitate, and platelets for DIC.

    D. Her smear should be evaluated for microangiopathic features, and, if present, she should be treated with emergent therapeutic plasma exchange daily until she demonstrates recovery or improvement of her counts.

338.

A 60-year-old woman with systemic lupus erythematosus is found to be anemic on routine testing. She is asymptomatic and denies any recent lupus symptoms.

Laboratory:

Hemoglobin	9.5 mg/dL (normal 13–16 mg/dL)
Reticulocyte count:	1.2% (0.2–2%)
MCV	86 (normal 76–100)
RDW	12 (9–14.5)
Serum iron	28 (normal 60–160 μg/dL)
TIBC	198 (normal 250–460)
% Fe sat	15% (normal 15–55%)
Ferritin	400 (normal 14–186)

The cause of her anemia is most likely which of the following?

A. Iron deficiency
B. B_{12} deficiency
C. Anemia of chronic disease
D. Sickle cell disease
E. Lupus anticoagulant

339.

Jason Banks is a 17-year-old with a history of prolonged bleeding episodes and epistaxis for many years. He presents to the Emergency Department with a particularly difficult epistaxis to control. He never has had a workup.

Testing is done and the following lab results are noted:

PT normal
aPTT 55 seconds (control 34 seconds)
CBC is normal with normal platelets
Bleeding time is prolonged
Factor VII levels are normal
RIPA (platelet aggregation in response to ristocetin) is abnormal

Which of the following is most likely diagnosis?

A. von Willebrand disease
B. Factor XIII deficiency
C. Factor VII deficiency
D. Bernard-Soulier syndrome
E. Vitamin K deficiency

340.

A 67-year-old man presents with increasing weakness and easy bruising. He has been healthy most of his life, except for a myocardial infarction 7 years ago. He had angioplasty without complication and has been doing well.

Physical Examination:
      HEENT: Pale conjunctiva, PERRLA, EOMI
      Throat: Clear
      Neck: Supple, without masses
      Heart: RRR without murmurs, rubs or gallops
      Lungs: CTA
      Abdomen: Marked splenomegaly
      Extremities: Scattered petechiae

Laboratory:
      WBC   1,800 with 60% polys
      Hemoglobin   7.8 mg/dL
      Platelets   74,000

A bone marrow aspiration is attempted, but the hematologist is unable to aspirate the marrow—it is a "dry tap."

What is the most likely etiology of his disorder?

A. Chronic myelogenous leukemia (CML)
B. Acute lymphocytic leukemia (ALL)
C. Hairy cell leukemia
D. Hodgkin disease
E. Non-Hodgkin lymphoma

341.

A 35-year-old man presents with abdominal and low back pain. He notes that recently, his urine is darker than usual.

Physical Examination:
    Vital signs are stable without fever
    HEENT: PERRLA, EOMI
    Throat: Clear
    Heart: RRR without murmurs, rubs, or gallops
    Lungs: CTA
    Abdomen: He has normal active bowel sounds with no tenderness. There are no abnormal masses in his
        abdomen, and his spleen is not enlarged. No bruits are heard.
    Back: He has no costovertebral angle tenderness. No abnormalities noted.
    GU: Normal male external genitalia

Laboratory:
Urine dip stick is negative except for 3+ RBCs. Microscopic examination of the urine shows no RBCs.
Reticulocyte count is 6%. Haptoglobin level is 0.

Which of the following is the most likely diagnosis?

A. Cystic fibrosis
B. Hemoglobinopathy
C. AML
D. ALL
E. Paroxysmal nocturnal hemoglobinuria (PNH)

342.

A 60-year-old man presents to you with fatigue. His physical examination shows splenomegaly but otherwise is normal.

Laboratory:
WBC: 2,600 with 12% monocytes, 12% polys, 76% lymphocytes
HCT: 30%
Platelets: 85,000

A bone marrow aspirate and biopsy are done. The aspirate is dry and the biopsy is pending.

Based on the information so far, what is the most likely diagnosis?

A. Myelofibrosis
B. Multiple myeloma
C. Hairy cell leukemia
D. Chronic lymphocytic leukemia (CLL)
E. Chronic myeloid leukemia (CML)

343.

A 1-year-old boy bleeds significantly after a minor hernia repair. He is the firstborn male. Neither parent has a bleeding diathesis. Platelet count, bleeding time, PT, and aPTT are all **normal**. You think to yourself, why are they asking me about a 1-year-old? Because they like to, and this problem appears on the Boards frequently because it is the only bleeding problem with all these other things being normal.

What is the most likely diagnosis?

A. Factor XII deficiency
B. Factor VII deficiency
C. von Willebrand's disease
D. Factor XIII deficiency
E. Protein S deficiency

344.

Which of the following is associated with the Philadelphia chromosome, t(9,22)?

A. Chronic lymphocytic leukemia (CLL)
B. Chronic myelogenous leukemia (CML)
C. Acute myelogenous leukemia (AML)
D. Acute lymphocytic leukemia (ALL)
E. Chronic myelodysplastic syndrome X

345.

A 65-year-old man presents to your office complaining of fatigue. He has also had exertional dyspnea for 4 months but has not had any chest discomfort during this time period. His wife cooks 3 meals a day for him, and he has "a good steak" on a weekly basis.

Past Medical History: HTN x 30 years, currently on hydrochlorothiazide

Social History: Smokes 1 pack/day for 30 years; Drinks 1–2 six-packs of beer daily

Physical Examination: BP 180/70, HR 100, Temp 98.5, RR 15
HEENT: Anicteric sclera, PERRLA, conjunctiva are very pale, no cheilosis
Heart: RRR with II/VI systolic murmur heard in the past without change
Lungs: Coarse wheezing
Abd: Liver palpable and nontender; spleen tip not palpated

Exteriors: Mild clubbing noted of fingers

Laboratory:
WBC	3,500
Hematocrit	27%
Platelets	97,000
MCV	109

Reticulocyte count is 0.8%
Peripheral smear shows targeting of large red cells without a leukoerythroblastic picture
AST	75
ALT	55
LDL	Normal

What is the <u>most</u> likely etiology for his anemia?

    A. Dietary vitamin B_{12} deficiency
    B. Myelodysplastic syndrome
    C. Hemolysis
    D. Iron deficiency anemia
    E. Alcoholism

346.

You have followed a patient for the 12 years, since her radiation treatment for Hodgkin disease. She received an upper mantle irradiation for an apparent cure of her disease. At the time of her visit today, she complains of fatigue, hair loss, and weight gain.

Appropriate tests should include which of the following?

    A. Repeat CT scans of her chest and abdomen for disease assessment
    B. Chemistry panel with a calcium
    C. A thyroid panel
    D. Pulmonary function tests

347.

A bone marrow aspirate is done and then stained with peroxidase. See Figure 3 at back of book.

Which of the following is associated with the finding in Figure 3?

    A. Acute lymphocytic leukemia (ALL)
    B. Acute myelogenous leukemia (AML)
    C. Chronic lymphocytic leukemia (CLL)
    D. Chronic myelogenous leukemia (CML)
    E. Hairy cell leukemia

348.

A 70-year-old man presents with lymphadenopathy, organomegaly, and neuropathy. He feels poorly. You suspect that he may have Waldenström macroglobulinemia.

Which of the following is associated with this disorder?

    A. Most cases occur in young women.
    B. Purpura is common.
    C. Hyperviscosity syndrome is uncommon.
    D. IgA levels are elevated.
    E. Median survival is 35 years.

349.

A 40-year-old man presents with a history of recurrent fevers and bleeding gums. He has noted recently an increased tendency toward bruising and has lost 15 lbs unintentionally. He is admitted to the hospital with urosepsis, with *Klebsiella* identified as the organism. Because of other findings, a bone marrow biopsy is done and demonstrates a leukemic infiltrate. The leukemic cells show resistance to tartrate inhibition. Cytoplasmic projections are noted.

Based on your findings, which of the following is true?

    A. A splenectomy is curative.
    B. Neutropenia is uncommon.
    C. This disease is associated with defects in antibody production only.
    D. A cutaneous vasculitis may also appear in this condition.
    E. The finding of cytoplasmic projections is uncharacteristic for this disorder.

350.

A 28-year-old woman has been healthy her whole life. She presents to the Emergency Department with confusion and fever. Her boyfriend has noted this morning that she appeared to be yellow.

Past Medical History: Negative

SOCIAL HISTORY: Works as a waitress in a local pub, Judge Roy Bean's
    Doesn't smoke or drink alcohol

Family History: Negative

Review of Systems: Faint rash noted by boyfriend

Physical Examination:
        BP 105/70, RR 18, Temp 102° F, P 100
        HEENT: PERRLA, EOMI   Scleral icterus
        TMs: Clear
        Throat: Palatal petechiae
        Neck: Supple

Heart: RRR without murmurs or rubs
Lungs: CTA
Abdomen: Benign
Extremities: Scattered petechiae on her lower extremities

Laboratory:
Hematocrit: 27%
WBC: 12,000/μL with 88% neutrophils
Platelet count: 13,000/μL
Total bilirubin: 7 mg/dL
Direct bilirubin: 0.7 mg/dL
BUN: 68 mg/dL
Creatinine: 4.8 mg/dL
PT: 12 sec (normal)
aPTT: 32 sec (normal)
Peripheral smear: Fragmented red blood cells and nucleated red blood cells

The best initial therapy for this condition is which of the following?

    A. High-dose glucocorticoids
    B. High-dose aspirin therapy
    C. Low-dose aspirin therapy
    D. Plasmapheresis
    E. Splenectomy

351.

You are presented the following laboratory values on the Board examination:

PT is increased
aPTT is normal
Platelet count is normal

Which of the following deficiency or abnormality would be responsible for these results?

    A. Factor VIII deficiency
    B. Factor VII deficiency
    C. Factor X deficiency
    D. Factor XIII deficiency
    E. Anti-platelet antibody

352.

A 37-year-old woman requires a mechanical valve for severe aortic stenosis. She is started on warfarin and develops skin necrosis.

Which of the following deficiencies does she most likely have?

A. Factor VIII deficiency
B. Factor XIII deficiency
C. Protein C deficiency
D. Antithrombin III deficiency
E. Factor V deficiency

353.

A 21-year-old African-American man comes in for a pre-insurance physical. His history and physical examination are normal. Routine laboratory is sent at the request of the insurance company and returns as follows:

WBC: 7,600/mm^3 with normal differential
Hemoglobin   17.0 mg/dL
MCV   66 fL

You order a hemoglobin electrophoresis, and it is normal.

Which of the following explains his laboratory finding of a low MCV?

A. Sickle cell trait
B. Sickle β-thalassemia
C. β-thalassemia trait
D. α-thalassemia trait
E. Sickle C disease

354.

You begin therapy on a patient who has pernicious anemia. You begin vitamin B$_{12}$ supplementation.

Which of the following electrolyte abnormalities should you be concerned about during the initial weeks of therapy?

A. Hypocalcemia
B. Hypercalcemia
C. Hypokalemia
D. Hyperkalemia
E. Hypernatremia

355.

A 50-year-old woman on chronic dialysis has anemia. She has had various studies evaluating this anemia. Iron deficiency and other vitamin deficiencies have been ruled out. It is thought that she has anemia of chronic disease.

Which of the following was most likely in her iron studies workup?

A. Serum iron was low, TIBC was high.
B. Serum iron was high, TIBC was low.
C. Serum iron was low, TIBC was low or normal.
D. Serum transferrin was high.
E. Bone marrow iron stores were low.

356.

Glucose-6-phosphatase deficiency (G-6PD) is fairly common.

Which of the following statements about G-6PD deficiency is true?

A. Drugs can trigger hemolysis.
B. It is usually autosomal dominant in transmission.
C. It is rare in African-Americans compared to Native-Americans.
D. G-6PD levels increase as the red cell ages.
E. Infections cannot induce hemolysis in a patient with G-6PD deficiency.

357.

A colleague of yours says that every time a patient has an elevated aPTT, you must be worried about a clinical bleeding disorder. You disagree and tell him that, actually, there is a disorder with an elevated aPTT, a normal PT, and no clinical bleeding noted.

What is this disorder?

A. Factor V deficiency
B. Factor VII deficiency
C. Factor VIII deficiency
D. Factor IX deficiency
E. Factor XII deficiency

358.

Which of the following may present with a normal PT, normal aPTT, but evidence of clinical bleeding and a prolonged bleeding time?

A. Factor VII deficiency
B. Factor VIII deficiency
C. Factor XII deficiency
D. von Willebrand disease
E. Factor V deficiency

ONCOLOGY

359.

Neurofibromatosis-2 is associated with which type of CNS tumors?

A. Optic gliomas
B. Giant cell tumors
C. Medulloblastoma
D. Hemangioblastoma
E. Vestibular schwannoma

360.

An 18-year-old male presents to your office with a 3-week history of left ankle pain. He just returned from a ski trip but was having pain before he left for the trip. He denies trauma to his ankle. He has had no fever, headache, vomiting, diarrhea, or cold symptoms. Review of systems is negative. Past medical history is significant for mild asthma.

On physical exam, he has swelling and tenderness over the anterior distal tibia. It hurts to bear weight. There is decreased range of motion.

X-ray reveals a tumor with both sclerotic and lytic changes with no definite transition between good bone and tumor. There is also elevated periosteum (Codman triangle).

You make the diagnosis.

Further evaluation should include all of the following except:

A. CT of the brain
B. CT of the lungs
C. MRI of the primary site
D. Bone scan
E. CBC

361.

A 60-year-old with a 90-pack year history of cigarette smoking presents to your office with hemoptysis and shortness of breath. A CXR reveals a cavitary lung nodule that is squamous cell by biopsy. He undergoes resection of the nodule. One year later, he presents with abdominal pain and constipation. His serum calcium is 19.

Appropriate next steps in his management include all of the following except:

A. Vigorous hydration with NS
B. Bisphosphonate treatment
C. CT chest
D. Phosphorus supplementation
E. Diuresis

362.

A 33-year-old woman presents to discuss options for breast cancer prevention. Her family history is positive for breast cancer as shown in this diagram.

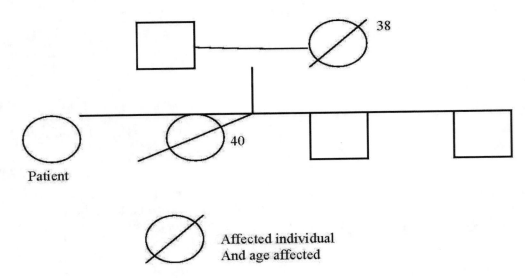

Patient

Affected individual
And age affected

Which of the following would be appropriate to tell her?

A. Tell her not to worry; her risk of breast cancer is the same as that for any other woman.
B. Tell her bilateral mastectomy will prevent any possibility for breast cancer.
C. Tell her to start mammograms at age 50 and have one done every other year.
D. Tell her the risk is increased at least 3-fold that of normal, and she should have testing for *BRCA-1* and *BRCA-2* genes.

363.

A 45-year-old finds a breast mass by self-exam. Mammogram is unable to locate the mass, and the study is read as normal. An exam by you confirms a 1-cm mass in the upper outer quadrant of the right breast. There is no palpable axillary adenopathy and she feels fine.

The appropriate next step would be which of the following?

A. Repeat self-exam every month and call if mass changes
B. Repeat mammogram in 6 months
C. Order a CA-125 level
D. Ultrasound followed by biopsy if solid
E. Simple mastectomy

364.

A 50-year-old postmenopausal woman finds a breast lump. Ultrasound and mammography confirm a suspicious 3-cm mass. A core biopsy is positive for infiltrating ductile carcinoma. A lumpectomy and axillary node dissection are done. The cancer is 3 cm with 2 positive axillary nodes. ER and PR receptors are negative. Her-2-Neu staining is negative.

You should recommend which of the following?

A. Close follow-up with an exam every month
B. Repeat surgery with conversion to a modified radical mastectomy
C. Local radiation therapy
D. Local radiation therapy followed by adjuvant chemotherapy
E. Local radiation therapy plus tamoxifen for 5 years

365.

A 60-year-old woman presents with increasing abdominal girth and shortness of breath. Physical exam reveals ascites, and a pelvic ultrasound reveals a right-sided adnexal mass.

Which of the following is <u>not</u> correct?

A. There is a > 85% likelihood the mass is a germ cell tumor.
B. There is increased risk of this malignancy with *BRCA-1* and *BRCA-2* abnormalities.
C. Treatment should include TAH/BSO with omentectomy, gross tumor resection, and biopsies of all serosal surfaces.
D. CA-125 should be ordered.
E. Most ovarian tumors are diagnosed with advanced-stage disease.

366.

Which of the following is true?

A. Testicular cancer is germ cell in origin > 95% of the time.
B. αFP and β-HCG may be elevated in pure seminoma.
C. αFP is secreted only by testicular tumors.
D. Most testicular germ cell tumors are associated with an isochromosome 15p.
E. Treatment for testicular cancer should include a transscrotal orchiectomy.

367.

A 50-year-old African-American male is seen in your office for his routine health maintenance exam. He asks what you recommend for prostate screening.

Which of the following should you tell him?

A. Screening is not recommended by the American Cancer Society.
B. Screening should include a transrectal U/S yearly.
C. A PSA and alkaline phosphatase should be checked every 2 years.
D. A bone scan and PSA should be done yearly.
E. A PSA and digital rectal exam should be done annually according to the American Cancer Society but is not routinely recommended by the USPSTF.

368.

A 28-year-old woman has a routine gynecologic evaluation. A Pap smear is done and returns with a diagnosis of low-grade squamous intraepithelial lesion. A biopsy reveals CIN II.

Which of the following statements is true?

A. No further treatment is required for CIN II.
B. A risk factor for cervical cancer is sexual abstinence.
C. HPV is associated with the development of cervical cancer (especially subtypes 16 and 18).
D. Appropriate next therapy would be hysterectomy.

369.

Which of the following statements is true?

A. IL-2 therapy is not associated with capillary leak syndrome.
B. GM-CSF is not associated with capillary leak syndrome.
C. ATRA (all-trans-retinoic acid) comes from the yew tree.
D. Alkylating agents (such as nitrogen mustard) cause infertility.
E. Carboplatin therapy causes more nausea and more nephrotoxicity than cisplatin.

370.

A true statement about bone marrow transplants includes which of the following?

A. Allogeneic transplant involves use of the patient's own bone marrow.
B. Autologous transplant involves use of a donor marrow.
C. Syngeneic transplant involves marrow donation from a twin.
D. Chronic myelogenous leukemia (CML) is never treated with bone marrow transplant.
E. Aplastic anemia is always treated with bone marrow transplant.

371.

A 56-year-old African-American man presents to your office with a three-month history of fatigue. He denies any other complaints and has no chronic past medical history. His physical exam is unremarkable.

Laboratory:
Hemoglobin 7.5   Total protein 10.0

Hematocrit 28%   Albumin 2.6
WBC 4,500   Globulins 7.4
Platelets 450,000

You strongly suspect a diagnosis of multiple myeloma, so you order which of the following set of tests?

A. Bone scan, urine protein electrophoresis, chemistries
B. Bone marrow aspirate and biopsy
C. Bone scan, serum protein electrophoresis
D. Immunofixations, quantitative immunoglobulins
E. Serum and urine electrophoresis, LDH, beta-2-microglobulin

---

372.

A patient is referred to your office by your family medicine colleague for evaluation and discussion regarding treatment options for chronic lymphocytic leukemia (CLL). The patient is a 42-year-old Caucasian male in relatively good health. He presented two months ago with lymphadenopathy and was noted to have a lymphocytosis. This was confirmed on a separate occasion and is persistent in all labs available.

He denies any systemic symptoms and specifically has had no fever, chills, or night sweats. His physical exam confirms bilateral cervical adenopathy measuring 2–3 cm. He has no other adenopathy and no organomegaly.

Laboratory:

2 months ago (at diagnosis)   At time of consultation
Hemoglobin: 12   Hemoglobin: 11.5
Hematocrit: 35   Hematocrit: 35
WBC: 125,000   WBC: 100,000
  Segs: 3%   Segs: 5%
  Lymphs: 97%   Lymphs: 95%
Platelets: 175,000   Platelets: 200,000

The most appropriate information for you to relate to the patient includes which of the following?

A. He has stage II disease and requires immediate therapy. His long-term prognosis is less than one year.
B. He has stage I disease and requires no immediate therapy. His long-term prognosis is excellent, and he should have a normal life expectancy.
C. He has stage I disease and requires no immediate therapy. His treatment options in the future include melphalan and prednisone versus consideration for a bone marrow transplant. His long-term prognosis is five to seven years with standard treatment.
D. He has stage IV disease and requires immediate therapy. His long-term prognosis is less than one year.
E. He was incorrectly diagnosed and has infectious mononucleosis.

373.

You are asked to see a patient in consultation at the hospital. The patient is a 22-year-old Caucasian female admitted for exploratory laparotomy for abdominal pain. She has had progressive pain and increasing abdominal girth for 2 months. She denies any systemic symptoms such as fever, chills, or night sweats. She has lost about 10 pounds over the last 2 months because she has been unable to eat as much as usual.

Her physical exam reveals a young female in no distress. She has no pathologic findings—other than a soft flow murmur at the upper left sternal border and obvious abdominal distention. Her liver is not palpable, but her spleen extends into the pelvis on the left. It is firm and only mildly tender.

Laboratory:

Hemoglobin 10
Hematocrit 29%
Uric Acid 15.3
LDH 600
WBC 256,340   LAP 2 (normal 78–106)
  segs 39%   HLA typing A1, A–, B3, B35, Dr1, Dr13
  bands 8%
  myelocytes 20%
  metamyelocytes 5%
  eosinophils 10%
  basophils 15%
  blasts 3%

Appropriate management now would include which of the following?

  A. Leukodepletion since the WBC count is > 100,000
  B. Hydration and treatment with appropriate antibiotics for a leukemoid reaction
  C. Intravenous induction chemotherapy for acute leukemia
  D. HLA typing of siblings with immediate BMT if a donor is available
  E. Discussion of treatment options to include hydroxyurea, alpha-interferon, and combination therapy with alpha-interferon plus ara-c

---

374.

A 70-year-old male smoker presents with severe back pain and pain in the pelvic girdle. X-ray shows osteoporosis of the spine. Labs: WBC 6,000, HCT 26, calcium 12, bone scan: negative.

What is the most likely diagnosis?

  A. Metastatic prostate cancer
  B. Prolonged corticosteroid use
  C. Metastatic lung cancer
  D. Multiple myeloma
  E. Avascular necrosis

375.

Muffin Man Forrest is a 74-year-old man diagnosed 3 years ago with poorly differentiated adenocarcinoma of the prostate. Staging at that time revealed no evidence of extraprostatic spread. He underwent radiation therapy because he did not want to lose his ability to have sex. Until recently, he has done well. Today, he presents with complaints of severe pain in his left hip. Physical examination shows marked pain with passive and active movement of the hip joint. No other abnormalities are found on physical examination.

Laboratory:
Prostate-specific antigen is elevated.
Bone scan shows new areas of uptake in the pelvis and ribs.

Today, he again says he would like to forego an orchiectomy if possible. He is willing to change his mind, he says, if it will significantly improve his quality of life or chance for survival.

The most appropriate therapy for him is which of the following?

A. Biopsy one of the bony lesions first before making any decisions.
B. Perform an orchiectomy since it will improve survival.
C. Administer cisplatin.
D. Perform an orchiectomy and administer cisplatin because the combination will improve survival.
E. Administer leuprolide and flutamide.

376.

A 31-year-old man presents for a routine examination. He has no specific complaints. He is a new patient.

Past Medical History:
Negative and his only medication is a multivitamin. He doesn't smoke but does drink an occasional glass of wine on the weekend.

Family History:
He notes that his father had colon cancer at age 43. His brother, who is 30-years-old, recently had a colonoscopy, at which time polyps were removed.

Which of the following is the best plan of action?

A. Colonoscopy now
B. Flexible sigmoidoscopy now—combined with fecal occult blood testing every year and a colonoscopy at age 40
C. Colonoscopy at age 50
D. Air contrast barium enema now

377.

A 40-year-old woman was recently diagnosed with malignant melanoma. She says that her grandmother died of malignant melanoma. She has a 0.7 mm diameter, irregularly-shaped melanotic lesion on the left side of her abdomen. A biopsy reveals the lesion extends to a 0.6 mm depth.

What is the best treatment for her?

A. Excise the lesion with a 1 cm tumor-free border.
B. Excise the lesion with a 3 cm tumor-free border and place her on chemotherapy.
C. Excise the lesion with a 3 cm tumor-free border.
D. Excise the lesion with a 5 cm tumor-free border.
E. Excise the lesion with a 0.7 cm tumor-free border.

378.

A 52-year-old woman presents for a routine physical examination. She has not had a mammogram so you schedule one for her. Her breast examination is otherwise normal. The mammogram shows a single small cluster of microcalcifications in the upper-outer quadrant of the left breast that is clinically nonpalpable.

What should the next step in her management be?

    A. No further evaluation is needed
    B. Fine-needle aspirate
    C. A mastectomy
    D. A needle-localized excisional biopsy
    E. A modified radical mastectomy

379.

Each condition below is associated with an increased risk of cancer of the esophagus, but one doesn't belong as a cause for, specifically, squamous cell carcinoma. (Think Sesame Street … one of these things isn't like the others ….)

Which one is <u>not</u> associated with increased risk of squamous cell carcinoma but is associated with adenocarcinoma of the esophagus?

    A. Achalasia
    B. Smoking
    C. Tylosis
    D. Alcoholism
    E. Barrett esophagus

380.

A 45-year-old pre-menopausal woman is diagnosed with breast cancer. She has staging done and the following are noted:

- Tumor was 0.5 cm.
- All nodes were negative.
- No distant metastases were noted.

In staging, she underwent a modified radical mastectomy because of pre-operative concerns of nodal involvement, which turned out to be just reactive lymph tissue.

Based on her staging and findings, what is the next appropriate therapy?

    A. Chemotherapy with anthracyclines and cyclophosphamide
    B. Hormonal therapy with trastuzumab
    C. Chemotherapy as above followed by hormonal therapy
    D. Radiation therapy
    E. No further therapy

381.

A 55-year-old man has a newly discovered testicular mass. He has a history of cryptorchidism as a child that was repaired at 3 months of age. Otherwise, he has been healthy without problems or symptoms. His testicular mass is painless.

Which of the following is <u>not</u> true regarding testicular cancer?

A. Most present as painless masses.
B. In men over 50, the testicular mass is more likely to be a seminoma than other types of tumor.
C. Abdominal cryptorchidism is a greater risk factor than inguinal cryptorchidism.
D. Patients with Klinefelter syndrome with mediastinal germ cells are at higher risk of developing testicular carcinoma.
E. Testicular ultrasound is indicated for a painless mass or one that does not resolve after several weeks.

382.

Which of the following chemotherapeutic agents is most commonly associated with renal toxicity?

A. 5-fluorouracil
B. Methotrexate
C. Vincristine
D. Vinblastine
E. Cisplatin

383.

Which of the following statements is <u>false</u> regarding basal cell carcinoma?

A. Basal cell carcinoma development is related to sun exposure.
B. Basal cell carcinoma cannot be inherited.
C. Basal cell carcinomas are locally aggressive.
D. Basal cell carcinomas are uncommonly seen in black skin.

384.

A 45-year-old man has lost thirty pounds in the last 8 weeks unintentionally. In addition, he was found to have velvety hyperpigmented plaques about his neck, axillae, mouth, breast, and groin. A diagnosis of acanthosis nigricans was made.

Assuming he has a neoplasm, which organ is the most likely site of the primary tumor?

A. Lung
B. Bladder
C. Prostate
D. Stomach

385.

A 36-year-old woman presents with numerous basal cell carcinomas, palmar and plantar pits, and cysts of the jaw. The basal cell carcinomas are distributed over her face, neck, and back. Her father has the same condition.

The most likely diagnosis is which of the following?

    A. Tuberous sclerosis
    B. Neurofibromatosis
    C. Nevoid basal cell carcinoma syndrome
    D. Gardner syndrome

386.

A 66-year-old patient comes to your office and gives a history of squamous cell carcinoma of his back. He tells you that the surgeon said the diagnosis was "carcinoma *in situ*." He asks you what this means.

Which of the following should you tell him?

    A. The cancer cells were confined to the epidermis.
    B. The cancer cells went through the dermis but not through the fat.
    C. The cancer has already spread to other parts of his body.
    D. None of the above.

NEUROLOGY

387.

A 16-year-old quarterback is hit while playing in his high school football game. There is no loss of consciousness, but he can't remember what happened. He is able to walk off the field under his own power. He has never had a concussion before. You are the team physician, and the coach wants to know when his star quarterback can return to the game.

His exam is normal except for the amnesia, so which of the following is your response to the coach?

A. He is out of the current game but can return to play after 1 week if no symptoms at rest and exertion.
B. He can return to the game after 20 minutes if no symptoms other than the amnesia.
C. Immediate hospitalization.
D. He is out for the season.
E. He is out for 1 month at least.

388.

A 19-year-old woman comes to your office complaining of frequent severe headaches, usually on the right. They are usually unilateral, throbbing, and associated with photophobia and phonophobia. She denies associated rhinorrhea, watering eyes, or conjunctival erythema. Often, these will worsen at the time of her menses. She has had them for about 1 year. They began with a frequency of one per month, but now occur about two times a month. The headaches last 3–4 hours. She denies associated neurologic problems such as weakness or numbness. So far, she has taken only over-the-counter medications like acetaminophen and ibuprofen. Both medicines will partially relieve her headache. There is a positive family history (in her mother and a maternal aunt) of similar headaches.

Physical Exam: She is average weight, and her general physical exam, neurological exam, and routine laboratories are normal.

Which of the following is the most likely diagnosis?

A. Migraine headache
B. Cluster headache
C. Tension headache
D. Pseudotumor cerebri
E. Intracranial tumor

389.

A 50-year-old man comes to the office with "clumsiness." This has been getting worse gradually over the past few weeks. At first, it involved the right foot. Later, he noticed problems in both feet and was "tripping over" his own feet. In the past week, he has noticed a change in his voice: It now sounds more "nasal." He denies recent infections. He has had no fever, chills, nausea, or vomiting.

On examination, he has a "nasal" sounding voice, but his speech is fluent. Naming and repetition are excellent. He has weakness of the legs more so than the arms. He has hyperreflexia.

Which of the following is the most likely diagnosis?

A. Huntington disease
B. Amyotrophic lateral sclerosis (ALS or Lou Gehrig disease)
C. Brain tumor in the dominant hemisphere
D. Herpes encephalitis

390.

A 44-year-old man comes to the Emergency Department with quickly worsening weakness of both arms and legs. Four days ago, he had low back pain. Two days ago, he noticed weakness of both legs. Initially, he had difficulty only when climbing stairs, but now he has trouble walking. Yesterday, the weakness spread to both arms. He denies bowel or bladder dysfunction. He denies recent trauma. He had an upper respiratory infection about two weeks ago. There is no family history of neurologic disease. He denies risk factors for HIV.

Physical Exam: He is awake, alert, and articulate. He has normal cranial nerves. He has 4/5 weakness in the upper and lower extremities bilaterally. The weakness is more pronounced in the distal extremities. Reflexes are 1+ in the arms. They are absent in the legs. Toes are downgoing bilaterally. There is no sensory level. There are no signs of cerebellar involvement.

Which of the following is the most likely diagnosis?

A. Guillain-Barré syndrome
B. Chronic inflammatory demyelinating polyneuropathy (CIDP)
C. Polyneuropathy
D. Transverse myelitis
E. Myasthenia gravis

391.

A 32-year-old man is brought in by his friends to the ED in a coma. The only available history is that he was found in the park by a jogger. His exam shows an obese, poorly developed man who is disheveled in appearance. He does not respond to noxious stimuli. He has bilateral pinpoint pupils. He does not smell of alcohol. There is no evidence of IV drug use.

What is the most likely cause of the patient's coma?

A. Brainstem infarct
B. Overdose (opiates)
C. Large middle cerebral artery infarct
D. Nonketotic hyperosmolar coma
E. Diabetic ketoacidosis

392.

A 49-year-old publishing magnate presents with complaint of severe stabbing headaches. "It feels like an ice-pick in my skull." When he gets the headaches, he also notes occasional lacrimation and nasal congestion. His headaches develop over 5–10 minutes and then last from 20 minutes to 2 hours. He reports lately he has had them 2–3 times daily and had similar episodes last year that lasted 8 weeks. These episodes seem to occur around a Board review conference.

What type of headaches does he seem to have?

A. Tension headache
B. Migraine headache
C. Cluster headache
D. Simple headache
E. Headache due to pseudotumor cerebri

393.

A 68-year-old woman presents with a left arm tremor. She has had the tremor for about 3 years and recently was noticed to have developed a side-to-side head tremor as well. Her tremor worsens when she performs movements that involve her bringing her hand to her face, such as smoking or drinking coffee. Of note is that if she drinks beer, the tremor seems to improve.

Which of the following is the likely etiology?

A. Parkinson disease
B. Myasthenia gravis
C. Benign essential tremor
D. Gilles de la Tourette syndrome
E. Huntington disease

394.

A 25-year-old woman presents with worsening weakness in her lower extremities. She denies headache, nausea, or vomiting. She has not had any significant illness except for a "stomach" flu 2 weeks ago. With this she had diarrhea for several days, but it has resolved.

Physical Examination:
HEENT: PERRLA, EOMI
                No cranial nerve abnormalities
Neck: Supple
Heart: RRR without murmurs, rubs, or gallops
Lungs: CTA
Abdomen: + BS, soft, non-tender
Extremities: No cyanosis, clubbing, or edema

Neurological Exam:
Marked weakness bilaterally over her lower extremities from the hip flexors down. She can barely lift her legs off the bed when in a lying position. Reflexes are absent in her lower extremities, and the brachioradialis reflex in her upper extremity is diminished bilaterally. Biceps tendon reflex appears to be intact.

Lumbar puncture is done and shows only an elevated protein. Special studies are pending.

The next day on examination her upper extremities are also becoming weak, and she has had some difficulty with breathing.

Which of the following is the best therapy to begin at this point?

    A. Plasmapheresis
    B. 5 mg of prednisone
    C. Await ANA before proceeding with further therapy
    D. Start interferon-alpha therapy
    E. Start interferon-beta therapy

395.

A 14-year-old lethargic girl is brought to the ED. Her mom reports the daughter has had recent nausea, vomiting, and abdominal pain. There is no recent fever, adenopathy, or malaise. On exam, she is quite sleepy, and has rapid, deep respirations. You think she might have a fruity smell to her breath.

What is the most likely cause of her altered mental status?

    A. Hypoglycemia
    B. Hyperosmolar state
    C. Ketoacidosis
    D. Pancreatitis
    E. Hypercalcemia

396.

A 56-year-old comatose obese woman is brought to the ED by her husband. She has had several days of headache and has been "sleepy." On the day of admission, she became unresponsive. On exam, she has hyperreflexia on the left (arm and leg), spasticity in the left upper and lower extremity, and seems to withdraw from painful stimuli, less well on the left. There is no atrophy or fasciculations of the muscles in the left arm or leg. Funduscopic exam shows bilateral papilledema; the right pupil is large and unreactive, while the left is midpoint and reacts to light.

What is the most likely cause of her coma?

    A. Ketoacidosis
    B. Pseudotumor cerebri
    C. Normal pressure hydrocephalus
    D. Hypercalcemia
    E. CNS tumor

397.

A 23-year-old woman comes to your office complaining of a unilateral throbbing headache that was preceded by "seeing flashing lights." The headache worsened over a 60-minute period, has been present for three hours, and seems to be getting better. The headache is severe, a "9/10." She is nauseous and had vomited. She says that the headache is worse if she sees bright lights or hears loud noises. She has had this type of headache since her early teens and has them two to four times per year. On examination, she has no weakness or numbness. There is no papilledema on funduscopic examination. Serum tests are normal.

Which of the following would you recommend for treatment?

A. Sumatriptan
B. Divalproex sodium/valproate
C. Propranolol
D. Verapamil
E. Amitriptyline

398.

A 68-year-old man is brought to your office by a family member (his daughter) due to a gradually worsening problem with short-term memory over the past 2–3 years. Further questioning identifies worsening urinary incontinence as well. His exam shows a mildly disheveled man in no distress. He has no focal neurological deficits. The funduscopic exam is negative for papilledema. His gait is magnetic.

Which of the following is the most likely diagnosis?

A. Alzheimer's dementia
B. Multi-infarct dementia
C. Normal pressure hydrocephalus (NPH)
D. Creutzfeldt-Jacob disease
E. Parkinson's disease

399.

An 80-year-old former nurse has been having gradually worsening short-term memory for 3 years. On neurological exam, she is pleasant but has difficulty naming objects such as a stethoscope. She has trouble following complex commands. There is no focal weakness or numbness. There has been no incontinence, and her gait is slow but normal. There is no resting tremor, masked facies, or festinating gait.

What pathologic findings would you be likely to see at autopsy?

A. Neurofibrillary tangles
B. Senile plaques
C. Granulovacuolar degeneration
D. All of the choices are correct
E. None of the choices are correct

400.

A 62-year-old man is brought to the ED due to worsening mental status. When the family is questioned, the family describes a worsening of cognition over the past 4–6 weeks. As he has worsened, he has had quick jerk-like movements of the extremities. On examination, he has myoclonus in both arms (the jerks); these are precipitated by sudden noises. In addition, he has bilateral spasticity, and hyperreflexia. He is quite confused and is oriented to person and month only.

What is the most likely diagnosis?

A. Alzheimer's dementia
B. Pick's disease
C. Hepatic encephalopathy
D. Creutzfeldt-Jacob disease (CJD)
E. Huntington's disease

401.

A 40-year-old woman comes to your office with complaints of gradually worsening memory. Her husband states that she has become irritable and "difficult to live with" over the past 9–12 months. There has been no fever, malaise, or neck stiffness. Her mother died at a young age of "something neurological." On examination, she has quick jerks in both arms and face.

Which of the following is the most likely diagnosis?

A. Sydenham chorea
B. Herpes encephalitis
C. Huntington disease
D. Creutzfeldt-Jacob disease
E. Infarct of the subthalamic nucleus

402.

A 35-year-old woman presents with intense, sudden vertigo that causes her to feel very nauseous. She notices muffled hearing and ringing in the ears. Over the next few hours, the episode resolves. On further questioning, she describes several other episodes in her life, beginning at the age of 26. The attacks are not brought on by sudden head or body movements. There was no antecedent viral illness. She denies other neurological symptoms.

What is the most likely diagnosis?

A. Cerebellopontine angle tumor
B. Benign positional vertigo
C. Acute vestibulitis
D. Ménière disease
E. Cerebellar infarct

403.

A 17-year-old woman is brought to the ED after having a witnessed generalized tonic-clonic seizure. She has a history of febrile seizures in childhood. On further questioning, you find that she has had episodic "staring" and unresponsiveness for the past two years. Observers report that she has lip smacking movements during the staring episodes. The episodes have been rare (about 4 per year), and she did not seek medical attention for these. She is otherwise well. Her exam is normal.

What would be the <u>least</u> effective medication to treat these events?

    A. Valproate
    B. Carbamazepine
    C. Ethosuximide
    D. Phenobarbital
    E. Lamotrigine

404.

A 67-year-old man is brought to the ED with a severe headache that he describes as the worst he has ever experienced. He has been feeling unwell for the past day and has a fever of 101.5° F. On exam, he is mildly sleepy and has neck stiffness. The remainder of his exam is without focal neurological signs.

CSF shows 100 WBC, all neutrophils (normal is less than 6 lymphocytes: there should be no neutrophils), a protein of 80 (normal is 20–45 mg/dL), and a glucose of 40 (normal is 50–80 mg/dL).

What is the most likely diagnosis?

    A. Bacterial meningitis
    B. Viral meningitis
    C. Bacterial abscess
    D. Herpes encephalitis
    E. Toxoplasmosis

405.

A 19-year-old college student is brought to the ED after having a generalized tonic-clonic seizure. His roommate says that he has been sick for 2–3 days and describes a febrile illness, headache, and irritability. The patient is somnolent and poorly responsive in the ED. There are no focal neurological deficits on exam.

Which of the following is the most likely diagnosis?

    A. Bacterial meningitis
    B. Viral meningitis
    C. Bacterial abscess
    D. Subarachnoid hemorrhage
    E. Viral encephalitis

406.

If you suspect HSV encephalitis in a patient, which test is most <u>specific</u> in confirming the diagnosis?

    A. MRI brain
    B. CT brain
    C. Polymerase chain reaction (PCR) for HSV
    D. EEG

407.

A 20-year-old woman presents for evaluation of headaches. She has had headaches for the past 3 months, and they occur about 4 times a month. The headaches are extreme and involve the left side of her head. She reports maximum intensity behind her left eye. Her symptoms get worse with exercise.

Usually she will go into a quiet room with the lights off, and the headache will go away in 4 hours. On occasion her headaches are associated with nausea. She has noted "flashing lights" before some of the headaches have occurred.

A complete neurologic examination reveals no abnormalities.

Which of the following do you recommend?

    A. CT scan with contrast
    B. MRI
    C. CT scan without contrast
    D. MRA
    E. No imaging at this time

RHEUMATOLOGY

408.

A 19-year-old girl with a kidney transplant sees you for left knee pain of 3 weeks duration. She originally had renal failure as a result of focal segmental glomerulosclerosis with nephrotic syndrome that was treated with high doses of steroids for nearly one year. She underwent a cadaveric kidney transplant 5 years ago, and her creatinine has been stable at 1.9. She is maintained on mycophenolate mofetil, tacrolimus, and prednisone. There is no history of trauma. On exam of her knee you find no abnormality, but she clearly has a limp when she walks.

Your next step in evaluation of this patient would be?

- A. Arthrocentesis of the knee for possible occult infection
- B. Kidney biopsy for occult rejection
- C. NSAIDs for control of pain and inflammation
- D. Obtain a DEXA scan
- E. Obtain an MRI of the left hip and knee

409.

A 15-year-old male runner comes to your clinic with the complaint of left heel pain off and on for a month. He is on the track team and runs cross-country. There is no known injury to his foot. The pain occurs mainly when he first gets out of bed in the morning and when he runs. It is located on the medial aspect of the heel.

On physical exam, there is no redness, swelling, or significant tenderness. Gait is normal. There is no tenderness at the insertion of the Achilles tendon into the calcaneus.

What is the most likely diagnosis?

- A. Plantar fasciitis
- B. Sprain
- C. Fracture
- D. Achilles tendonitis
- E. Calcaneal apophysitis

410.

A 20-year-old man presents to clinic with back pain and stiffness. He has had these symptoms for about 8 months. In the beginning, he tried over-the-counter medications, but they did not help. His pain was initially in the lower back area and seemed to improve with exercise or movement. He has no radiation of the pain. He has had "itchy eyes" but seems to think these are normal with his allergies this time of year.

His physical examination is significant for slightly injected conjunctiva. He has a II/VI early diastolic murmur heard best at the 2nd left intercostal space. His musculoskeletal examination shows no active synovitis. He is tender over both of his sacroiliac joints but has normal lumbo-sacral movement. He has a negative leg-raising sign. He does not have psoriasis.

Which of the following should you do next to confirm the diagnosis?

    A. X-ray of the sacroiliac joints
    B. HLA-B27 serology
    C. Echocardiogram
    D. Chest x-ray
    E. Ophthalmology consult

411.

A 40-year-old woman presents for a follow-up appointment. Last month you evaluated her for complaints of persistent joint pains. At that time she had symmetrical swelling of her wrists, MCPs, and PIPs. You placed her on a nonsteroidal antiinflammatory agent that provided some relief, but she still has similar complaints. Her physical examination today is no different from last month's. An x-ray of the hands shows erosive synovitis in the MCP and PIP joints of both hands.

Which of the following is <u>not</u> consistent with a diagnosis of rheumatoid arthritis?

    A. Swelling of the wrist, MCPs, or PIPs for 6 weeks
    B. Erosive synovitis changes of her hands on x-ray
    C. Morning stiffness for longer than 45 minutes for 6 weeks
    D. Sacroiliitis
    E. Mononeuritis multiplex

412.

A 60-year-old man presents with complaints of left knee pain. He says that he has had chronic bilateral hip, knee, and shoulder pain for many months. These joints are usually "stiff" in the morning but improve after 20 minutes. His left knee became swollen 3 days ago and this is new. He cannot bear weight on this leg without severe pain in his knee. His physical examination shows a swollen, red, warm left knee. He has a palpable effusion of the affected knee. The neurological, vascular, and sensory functions of the knee area are intact.

You aspirate the knee and it shows 1,800 WBC/μL with 95% lymphocytes. No crystals or other abnormalities are noted.

What is the probable etiology of his left knee findings?

    A. Rheumatoid arthritis
    B. Gout
    C. Septic arthritis
    D. Pseudogout
    E. Degenerative joint disease

413.

Which of the following is the initial treatment for mild rheumatoid arthritis?

A. Prednisone
B. Gold salts
C. Aspirin
D. Cyclophosphamide
E. Methotrexate

414.

Which of the following synovial fluid findings is <u>most</u> consistent with gout?

A. Fluid, clear and viscous; WBC 400; no crystals
B. Fluid, cloudy and watery; WBC 7,500; no crystals
C. Fluid, dark brown and viscous; WBC 1,000; no crystals
D. Fluid, cloudy and watery; WBC 11,000; needle-like and strongly negatively birefringent crystals
E. Fluid, cloudy and watery; WBC 5,000; rhomboid in shape and weakly positively birefringent crystals

415.

A 74-year-old female presents to you with a 2-month history of bone pain, weight loss, and night sweats. She is very concerned by a red swelling over her left index finger. She has a history of NIDDM and coronary artery disease.

Physical Examination:
Well nourished and alert woman who appears her stated age. Neck supple. No lymphadenopathy. Mild splenomegaly is noted. Asymmetric Heberden and Bouchard nodes noted with erythema and profound tenderness over left second index DIP.

Laboratory:
ESR = 118, Hgb = 10.0, Creatinine = 2.4
Serum protein electrophoresis reveals a monoclonal spike.
Urine is positive for Bence-Jones protein.

What is the cause of her acute left finger symptoms?

A. Amyloid
B. Gout
C. Osteoarthritis
D. Pseudogout
E. Ochronosis

416.

A 60-year-old man presents with pain in his hip. He denies other symptoms except for occasional night sweats. His calcium is elevated.

Which of the following will have a normal bone scan?

    A. Fracture
    B. Osteomyelitis
    C. Multiple myeloma
    D. Osteoblastic type of malignancy
    E. Avascular necrosis

417.

A 50-year-old woman with complaints of joint pain for several months presents for evaluation. She reports that she has had morning stiffness for the last 3 months that lasts over an hour and gradually improves. She has had swelling of her wrists and PIP joints for about 2 months and some swelling in her knees for about 6 weeks.

Physical examination shows marked swelling of her wrists and PIP joints that is symmetrical. You note some nodules on the dorsum of her hands as well. Plain film x-rays of her hands show erosive synovitis.

Which of the following is her most likely diagnosis?

    A. Pseudoxanthoma elasticum
    B. Rheumatoid arthritis
    C. Osteoarthritis
    D. Ankylosing spondylitis
    E. Psoriatic arthritis

418.

A 70-year-old Caucasian man presents with a 3-month history of muscle pain, especially in his shoulders and pelvic girdle. He has severe morning stiffness on arising.

On physical examination no muscle atrophy is noted.
Upper extremities: No weakness noted
Lower extremities: No weakness noted

Laboratory:
ESR is 120 mm/hr; ANA is 1:40 with a speckled pattern.

Which of the following is the most likely diagnosis?

    A. Polymyositis
    B. Multiple myeloma
    C. Rheumatoid arthritis
    D. SLE
    E. Polymyalgia rheumatica

419.

A 50-year-old man presents with acute swelling of his first metatarsal joint. He admits to excessive alcohol intake and is on hydrochlorothiazide for hypertension. He is obese.

You tap the knee and discover urate crystals in the joint fluid.
Uric acid levels are normal.

What is the most likely diagnosis?

- A. Because of his age, alcohol intake, and normal uric acid levels, pseudogout is more likely.
- B. Because of his age, alcohol intake, and normal uric acid levels, hemochromatosis is more likely.
- C. Gout has definitively been diagnosed.
- D. Without knowing the birefringence, unable to assess if this is pseudogout or gout.
- E. Septic arthritis is most likely.

420.

A 30-year-old African-American woman presents with new onset of serositis. She has been well except for a cardiac arrhythmia, which required her to be started on a cardiovascular drug a few months ago. She is noted on exam to have serositis, but she has no evidence of renal or CNS involvement. She does not have a rash.

Which of the following is true about her condition?

- A. Anti-histone antibodies are rarely positive.
- B. Procainamide could have induced this.
- C. Rash is usually more common than serositis with this presentation.
- D. The absence of renal involvement in this case is unusual.
- E. Fever is uncommon.

421.

A 78-year-old woman comes to your office because of severe headache. She has also had muscle aches in her thighs, loss of appetite, malaise, and experiences jaw pain when eating or talking for a long period of time. On exam, she has no nuchal signs but does have tenderness over the temporal region. There are no focal findings on her neurological examination.

Which test will help to make a definitive diagnosis?

- A. Erythrocyte sedimentation rate (ESR)
- B. Temporal artery biopsy
- C. MRI of the brain
- D. CT of the brain
- E. Lumbar puncture

422.

A 47-year-old woman presents to her internist with painful swelling of her joints. Specifically, she has had problems with her finger joints, wrists, elbows, shoulders, knees, and feet, and complains of early morning stiffness lasting several hours. She is very concerned because her grandmother suffered from very bad RA. Her older sister has been diagnosed with apparent lupus. Her medical history is benign except for a history of HTN, which has been controlled with diuretics for several years. Her menses have become a little irregular of late. She is sleeping poorly and states that her energy levels have been almost "non-existent." She admits to significant stress, presently undergoing a divorce.

Exam reveals a healthy-appearing woman with BP 147/92, P 92, R 22, weight 212, height 5'6". She is not pale. Cardiorespiratory exam is benign. Abdomen is obese but no masses are appreciated. A complete MSK exam reveals no synovitis about the PIP or MCP joints. Grip strength is excellent. The wrists, elbows and shoulders all have a good ROM and no synovitis is detected. No effusions are noted in the knees and no crepitus. No metatarsalgia or clawing of the feet. Cutaneous exam is without psoriasis. She is tender on the lateral aspects of the shoulders and over the subtrochanteric areas bilaterally. She is tender in the lower lumbar areas and over the left anterior chest wall. As part of her workup, she is found to have a positive RF and ANA, and has a Sed rate of 9. Her hemoglobin is 12.7, WBC is 7.6, and platelet count is 212.

Which of the following statements is true?

A. She has RA and should begin methotrexate immediately.
B. She probably has SLE, and anti-dsDNA antibodies should be checked.
C. She has an overlap of RA and SLE.
D. She probably has fibromyalgia but should be monitored for the remote possibility of early RA.

423.

A 27-year-old female with seropositive erosive nodular RA currently receives methotrexate and infliximab (Remicade®) with good disease control. She calls your office because last night she saw a television show on the discovery channel about Jonas Salk and the history of vaccines.

Which vaccine should she not receive?

A. Tetanus toxoid
B. H1N1 influenza vaccine
C. Hepatitis B vaccine
D. Varicella vaccine
E. *Neisseria meningitidis* vaccine

424.

A 47-year-old female presents with symptoms of "grittiness" of her eyes and dryness of her mouth. She has had problems reading recently. She was recently seen by an ophthalmologist, who thought she might have early Sjögren's syndrome, and a Schirmer's test was apparently positive. Other than occasional pain in the wrists, she really has no joint problems. She denies rashes, SOB, cough, dysphagia or dysuria. She recently underwent a benign breast biopsy. Her family history is noncontributory.

On examination today, she is alert and oriented. Height 5'5", weight 112, P 76. She is not pale or jaundiced. The cardiorespiratory exam is benign. The abdomen has no masses. There is no lymphadenopathy. Complete musculoskeletal exam is negative. Cutaneous exam is benign. Exam of the oral mucosa reveals diminished salivary pool. Special investigations reveal her CBC to be normal. CMP is normal. ANA is strongly positive and the anti-SSA is positive.

This patient is __not__ at risk for which of the following?

A. Peripheral neuropathy
B. Renal tubular acidosis
C. Non-Hodgkin lymphoma
D. Barrett esophagus
E. Lymphocytic interstitial pneumonitis

425.

A 35-year-old male marathon runner with a history of GERD (successfully treated with a proton pump inhibitor) is referred for evaluation of 6 weeks of skin thickening involving his trunk and upper extremities but sparing his hands and fingers. This condition began after he completed a triathlon.

Which physical exam finding or laboratory abnormality would you expect this patient to have?

A. Raynaud phenomenon
B. Peripheral eosinophilia
C. Sclerodactyly
D. Positive ANA
E. Synovitis

426.

A 37-year-old African-American female presents with symptoms of fatigue. She is ordinarily used to exercising 5–6 times a week and recently has not been enjoying her light weight-lifting and yoga exercises. She feels short of breath and tired during exercise and has noticed some aching in her finger joints and her knees. In general, she has been in excellent health. Her weight is constant and she denies any fevers, night sweats or rashes. She has been waking up a little short of breath at night but blames this on some anxiety. She is presently going through a divorce.

On exam she is alert and oriented, well-nourished, and well-hydrated. Height 5'6", weight 127, BP 112/76, P 64. Cardiac exam is benign and respiratory tract reveals some crackles at both bases. There are no rashes. As part of her workup, she has a normal TSH, creatinine of 0.6, SGOT of 127 with the upper limit of normal being 35, and SGPT of 126 with upper limit of normal being 36. CK is 17,300 with the upper limit of normal being 160.

Which of the following autoantibodies is likely to provide the most significant insight into her disease process?

A. ANA
B. RF
C. C3 level
D. Anti-U1-RNP
E. Anti-Jo-1

427.

A 45-year-old female is referred from the Ophthalmology Clinic. She presented recently with retinal vasculitis with the venous system being more involved. A diagnosis of Behçet's had been considered because of a previous presentation with iritis several years prior to this. She also has a lengthy history of oral ulcers and had been diagnosed with complex oral aphthosis by a dermatologist several years ago. Two months ago she presented to her gynecologist with severe labial ulcerations. These have continued to be a problem over the past few months. She is not short of breath or coughing but is quite concerned about a new onset of an acne-like rash on her face and trunk. The joints of her fingers have become very painful. She underwent a subtotal thyroidectomy 18 months ago and is presently on thyroid replacement.

On exam, she is well nourished and well hydrated with T 97.8° F, BP 112/84. Cardiac and respiratory exam is benign. Oral mucosa reveals multiple aphthae. Genital exam revealed a 2x2 cm healing ulcer over the left labial area. Cutaneous exam is positive for a hyperpigmented acne-like rash over the face and chest. Investigations reveal a Sed rate of 37, RF and ANA negative, hemoglobin of 11.2, and WBC of 9.3.

Which of the following drugs would <u>not</u> be reasonable options for treating her condition?

   A. Thalidomide
   B. Methotrexate
   C. IV cyclophosphamide
   D. Colchicine

428.

A 37-year-old female with known lupus presents to the clinic with pain in her right deltoid area. This pain has become progressive over the past two months, to the point that it is waking her up at night. She has initiated a new exercise program and somehow thinks that this may be related. She is also typing in an uncomfortable position. The other joints have not been a problem. She denies any fever, weight loss, night sweats, rashes, or oral ulcers. Her energy levels are excellent. In the past she has had a malar rash as one of her manifestations and presented with synovitis of the PIP joints. She had minimal proteinuria but has never had nephrosis. Her ANA and anti-dsDNA had been strongly positive in the past. For her joint pain and rash, she had been on hydroxychloroquine sulfate for 18 months but discontinued this drug about two years ago per her rheumatologist's recommendation.

Exam showed the patient to be well-appearing and normotensive. No oral aphthae are noted. No lymphadenopathy. Cardiac and respiratory exam is benign. The left shoulder abduction is normal to 180 degrees, but she is able to abduct the right shoulder only to 70 degrees. There is no tenderness in the subacromial space.

Which of the following possibilities form part of her differential diagnosis?

   A. Avascular necrosis of the right shoulder
   B. Rotator cuff tendinopathy
   C. Rotator cuff tear
   D. Subacromial bursitis
   E. Acromioclavicular degenerative disease

429.

A 19-year-old male presents with low back pain and stiffness. These symptoms have been of gradual onset over the past six months. In general, he finds that a shower in the morning tends to make him feel less stiff, and once he starts walking around, the stiffness seems to disappear. There is no family history of consequence. His other peripheral joints have not been a problem, but more recently he has begun to notice some pain in the left groin area. There is no history of urethritis or of conjunctivitis. He has had no rashes. Otherwise, he has been in excellent health.

The patient is well-appearing. His peripheral joints are benign. Schober's test reveals 3 cm of movement. Cutaneous exam reveals no vasculitis, but some pitting is noticed on several nails and onycholysis of several others. Investigations reveal a sedimentation rate of 97, normal CBC and CMP, negative ANA and RF. X-ray of the lumbar spine reveals bilateral asymmetric SI joint sclerosis and narrowing. X-ray of the hips is normal.

Which would seem to be the drug of choice?

   A. Azulfidine
   B. Methotrexate
   C. Hydroxychloroquine sulfate
   D. Prednisone 60 mg qd
   E. An anti-TNF agent

430.

A 47-year-old male is seen on consultation in the ICU. He presented to the local ED short of breath and with hemoptysis three days prior to the initial consult. He arrested in the ED and required intubation and was transferred to the ICU. Oxygen demands were such that he was placed on extracorporeal membrane oxygenation (ECMO). He tolerated this well. The initial CXR revealed diffuse infiltrates bilaterally. Bronchoscopy revealed serosanguineous fluid, and visualization was generally poor. The family stated that he had been in excellent health except that he tended to drink 2–3 beers per night, occasionally more on the weekends.

Exam is generally benign without vasculitis; no rashes were detected. No obvious joint swelling or synovitis was noted. He was found to have a sedimentation rate of 63 and a positive ANA. U/A revealed two red cells per high-powered field. There were some red cell casts.

Which of the following tests are likely to be positive?

   A. c-ANCA
   B. p-ANCA
   C. Anti-GBM antibodies
   D. All of the choices are correct
   E. None of the choices is correct

431.

A 68-year-old woman with a history of Sjögren syndrome for 7 years manifested by intermittent bilateral parotid swelling, arthralgias, positive anti-Ro antibody, and a positive lip biopsy. She experiences significant sicca symptoms and recently read a report on the Internet about prednisone for the treatment of Sjögren's.

Which of the following statements about treatment of sicca symptoms is correct?

A. Steroids are ineffective in treating sicca symptoms.
B. 30 mg/day is effective in treating sicca symptoms.
C. 1 mg/kg is effective in treating sicca symptoms, but the side effects will limit their usefulness.
D. Only dexamethasone is effective in treating sicca symptoms.
E. The combination of steroids and cyclosporine ophthalmic emulsion (Restasis®) is effective in treating sicca symptoms.

432.

A 57-year-old female with a 10-year history of rheumatoid arthritis comes to see you in your office for her routine follow-up visit. Her joints are fairly asymptomatic. She has not had any recent flare ups and is well pleased with her function. However, she is quite concerned with a new onset of low back pain, which has been present for about the past six weeks. There has been no trauma. She has no bowel or bladder incontinence. The pain does not radiate, and she denies any numbness or tingling of her legs. There is no lower extremity weakness. She does not ascend stairs with comfort. Her current therapy includes methotrexate 15 mg q week, prednisone 3 mg qd, from which she is attempting to taper herself, and occasional ibuprofen. She is also on hydrochlorothiazide 25 mg qd for mild HTN.

On exam she is alert, oriented, and well-nourished. BP 127/76, P 76 and regular. Joint exam reveals minimal second right MCP synovitis and 3rd left PIP synovitis but excellent grip strength. She has two small rheumatoid nodules over her left olecranon area. There is no crepitus of the knees, but there is mild metatarsalgia of both feet.

Which of the following is <u>incorrect</u>?

A. Her back pain is clearly part of her RA.
B. The possibility of an osteoporotic fracture exists.
C. She has unrelated mechanical back pain.
D. None of the choices are incorrect.

433.

A 69-year-old female with known HTN returns for follow-up. She has been previously non-compliant with her antihypertensive medication, citing financial constraints. She is meant to be on a combination of a thiazide and an ACE inhibitor, of which she has taken neither for the past two months. She has noticed occasional palpitations but no chest pain. Since her last visit five months ago, she has noticed pain in her feet. One of her sons has gout, and she is concerned that this is her problem. She wants to have her uric acid level checked today. She has some pain over the DIP joints, which has been present for several years. The right knee continues to be painful after walking one city block or so. She has had several episodes in which her feet have become swollen and is quite concerned about pain around the right ankle area. She denies the use of alcohol. She has noticed some polyuria and polydipsia.

On exam she is alert, well nourished, and well hydrated. BP 187/99, P 100, R 20. JVD is not elevated. Cardiac exam reveals an S_4, and the lungs are clear. Complete review of MSK exam reveals mild asymmetric Heberden and Bouchard nodes. There is crepitus of both knees noted. There is bilateral 4+ lower extremity edema noted. No tophi are noted. Her labs from that date reveal a WBC of 7.3, hemoglobin of 16.2, creatinine of 1.9, and uric acid level is 8.2 (upper limit of normal in that lab 8.0).

Which of the following is appropriate?

A. Compliance with her hypertensive medication should be discouraged.
B. The patient should be initiated on allopurinol 450 mg qd.
C. The drug of choice would be probenecid.
D. The patient is at risk for allopurinol hypersensitivity syndrome.

434.

A 27-year-old female with known lupus is brought into the ED by her concerned family. Over the past 2–3 days they have noticed that she has become increasingly somnolent, has complained of a low-grade headache, appears distracted, and seemingly has had some memory problems. In the past she has been diagnosed with lupus based upon a positive ANA, arthralgias, positive anti-dsDNA, positive anti-SM, and a mild thrombocytopenia ranging from 75–90,000. Occasionally she has had a sun-exposed rash. More recently, she has been quite well. She was last in the ED about three months ago, at which time she had mild right leg edema. This was thought to be related to a DVT, but Doppler proved to be negative. As part of that workup, she was found to be lupus anticoagulant positive. She is single, has never been married, and is not presently sexually active. She is not on any medications.

Exam reveals a somewhat somnolent and otherwise healthy-appearing female with BP 112/76, P 90. She is well-nourished and her neck is supple. MSK exam is negative. Cutaneous exam reveals mild livedo reticularis. CT scan of the head done in the ED is entirely normal. Sedimentation rate is 22, WBC is 3.9, hemoglobin is 10.8, and platelet count is 74,000. U/A is clear. CSF is entirely clear with normal protein and glucose and no cells noted.

Which of the following is the most likely explanation for her presentation?

A. CNS vasculitis
B. Aseptic meningitis
C. Lupus cerebritis
D. Cerebrovascular infarct which does not show up in CT scan but most likely would show up on MRI
E. Post-ictal state

435.

A patient is treated with prednisone 20 mg qd for what was thought to be CNS cerebritis as part of her lupus. Her prednisone dose was slowly tapered over two months. Approximately five months after this, she returns with a fairly sharp headache, mild joint pain, and a fever. She is complaining of left-sided weakness with her leg feeling weaker than the arm. She had gone to sleep the previous night feeling quite well except for a mild headache, but woke up at 4:00 a.m. with a fairly sharp headache and a sense of weakness on the left as described above. When seen in the ED, it was fairly apparent that she had a left hemiparesis. She had no other new findings of note. A repeat CT scan of the brain is entirely normal; this was done without any contrast. At this time, her WBC is 2.7, hemoglobin is 11.0, and platelet count is 62,000.

Which of the following is the most appropriate management at this stage?

A. Low-dose aspirin
B. Initiate IV heparin and schedule MRI of the brain
C. Solu-Medrol 1 gram IV for three consecutive days
D. IV cyclophosphamide q month

436.

Consider a 72-year-old woman with known mild osteoarthritis and HTN, who consistently takes a thiazide diuretic and occasional celecoxib 200 mg qd for hand and knee pain. She has otherwise been in excellent health. She is admitted for a right lower lobe pneumonia and prescribed IV antibiotics. On the third day of her admission, she presents with an acutely swollen, tender, and painful right knee. This is the first time that any joint has actually swollen to such an extent. There is no history of podagra. Her uric acid level has always been normal. There is no history of renal calculi.

On exam she is alert, well-oriented and well-hydrated. BP 162/76, T 99.7. MSK exam reveals asymmetric Heberden's nodes and a large right knee effusion. The right knee effusion is tapped.

Which of the following findings are most likely in this clinical setting?

    A. Positively birefringent crystals
    B. Negatively birefringent crystals
    C. Calcium oxalate crystals
    D. Synovial fluid that is a transudate with a WBC of 2,200

437.

A 23-year-old female presents to your office with an 18-month history of RA. She has recently moved across the country and is seeking care. Her previous rheumatologist had diagnosed her with RA based on positive RF, erosive arthritis, and nodules that developed soon after the onset of her disease process. Three months after the onset of her disease process, she was started on methotrexate, which was slowly increased up to 15 mg per week. At this dose, she developed oral aphthae. Her joints seemingly were well-controlled. When the dose was reduced to 12.5 mg a week, her oral aphthae disappeared but her joints were quite painful and she was not fully controlled. It was more or less at this stage that her husband was transferred to an area near your office. In the interim, her previous rheumatologist had placed her on prednisone 5 mg qd, which controlled her symptoms very well. She did not want to start any other therapy until she had settled down in her new environment. At this time, her joints are fairly inactive. The remainder of the systemic inquiry is negative. She has been married for almost 18 months and has no children. She is using an oral contraceptive. Both the patient and her husband are interested in having children within the next year or so.

On exam, she is alert and oriented. Cardiorespiratory exam is negative. MSK exam reveals bilateral symmetric PIP and MCP joint synovitis with left wrist tenosynovitis. Her right elbow has two small rheumatoid nodules. There is a small left knee effusion. Cutaneous exam is negative. Her ESR is 42, and hemoglobin is 10.7.

Based on her desire to have children, which of the following is the best recommendation?

    A. Continue methotrexate at the present dose but add a biologic agent and suggest that an eventual plan would be to taper her off of the methotrexate if possible
    B. Add leflunomide 20 mg qd
    C. Add hydroxychloroquine sulfate 200 mg bid
    D. Continue with her present therapy
    E. All of the choices are correct

438.

A 43-year-old woman with known scleroderma presents with symptoms of reflux. She has previously had intermittent episodes of dysphagia, but this is not presently a problem. The symptoms of reflux have become much more pronounced over the past two months. There are some financial constraints, and she cannot afford her PPI medication. Previously she has been noted to have severe episodes of Raynaud's with occasional ulcers on her fingers, which have been quite tender and painful. She gives no history of recent ulceration. Her BP has always been normal thus far. She has tried calcium channel blockers with limited success for her Raynaud's attacks. She is not short of breath or coughing and has no dysuria.

Exam reveals a somewhat thin-looking female, weight 103, height 5'5", BP 176/92, P 82. Cardiac exam reveals a fourth heart sound and the lungs are clear. The cutaneous exam reveals sclerodactyly with telangiectasia, particularly on the palms, face, and chest.

Which of the following is applicable to her case?

A. Her BP needs to be controlled with an ACE inhibitor; BP control and compliance needs to be emphasized to the patient.
B. Once her reflux symptoms are managed, she does not need to have a Doppler ECHO to estimate pulmonary pressures.
C. She should be placed back on calcium channel blockers after her reflux is controlled.
D. All of the choices are applicable.

439.

A 57-year-old female presents to your office with numbness and tingling of the right wrist and hand. This has been present for the past six weeks and seems to be somewhat worse at night. These symptoms are improved by flicking her wrist. She has no symptoms on the other side. Her general medical inquiry is entirely negative. She has no paresthesias in the lower extremities. She has never had DM or HTN and is not on any medications whatsoever. She is married, is a housewife, and has two children. She has been typing more on her computer recently.

On exam she is alert and oriented, well nourished, and well hydrated. BP 112/72, P 72. Cardiorespiratory exam is negative. MSK exam is negative. Neurological exam is negative, completely without any sensory or motor deficits.

Which of the following is the most likely diagnosis?

A. Ulnar neuropathy
B. Cervical disc degenerative disease
C. Median nerve entrapment
D. Brachial plexopathy

440.

A 42-year-old gentleman presents with severe headache and fever. He is seen in his local ED and is complaining of a slightly stiff neck. Meningitis is considered, and a CSF tap is completed, which is negative. CSF protein is normal. No white cells were found in the CSF. As part of the workup, a CT scan is completed in the ED and significant sphenoidal sinus enlargement and engorgement is noted. He has a history of a 15-pound weight loss over a six-week period prior to his admission. He has had significant headaches. In general, he has been in excellent health. He has never had sinusitis before, though he does remember having otitis media diagnosed by his primary care physician about eight weeks ago, treated with oral amoxicillin for seven days. He has also noted a rash over the anterior shins, which is non-itchy. This developed over the last two days. Over the past 24 hours, there has been some numbness and tingling of both lower extremities.

On exam, he is oriented but a little apathetic. T 102.3° F, BP 112/72, P 94. Neck is supple. Cardiac exam is negative and lungs reveal some coarse wheezing. The abdomen is soft with hepatosplenomegaly. Joint exam is negative. Cutaneous exam reveals a fine, erythematous, vasculitic lower extremity rash. Neurologic exam reveals no sensory or motor deficits. Investigations reveal a normal CXR. His hemoglobin is 9.8, WBC is 15.3, and platelet count is 276. His sed rate is 123, creatinine is 1.2, and U/A reveals 2+ RBCs with red cell casts.

Which of the following is most likely to provide a diagnosis?

A. ANA
B. c-ANCA
C. p-ANCA
D. Anti-dsDNA antibodies
E. Anti-SCL70

441.

A 59-year-old female presents with aching of the shoulders and buttocks. These symptoms have been present for the past two weeks. Her energy levels are poor, and she has been avoiding her usual water aerobics program due to lack of energy and simply not feeling good. Her joints have also been aching. She is in otherwise excellent health except for a previous history of hypothyroidism, for which she is on an appropriate thyroid replacement dose. Her endocrinologist told her two months ago that her TSH level was WNL. She has no history of headaches, rashes, or previous joint pain. Exam is entirely normal.

Which of the following statements apply to this patient?

A. She probably has polymyositis, and CK levels are more than likely to be elevated. She will require prednisone 60 mg qd for this presumed diagnosis. A muscle biopsy is not necessary.
B. It is most likely that her sed rate will be quite elevated. If this is found to be the case, her diagnosis is most likely that of polymyalgia rheumatica (PMR), and she should be initiated on prednisone 15 mg qd.
C. She probably has PMR. Her CRP will, in all likelihood, be extremely elevated. She should be started on prednisone 60 mg qd.
D. She most probably has fibromyalgia and should be started on a low dose of amitriptyline.

442.

A 62-year-old gentleman with known acromegaly and DM comes to see you for an acutely swollen right big toe. This is not the first such event, and he has had at least four similar events for which he has been seen in his local ED and diagnosed with gout. His joints have never been aspirated. On one other occasion he remembers the right elbow being painful and swollen, but this settled down on its own after 4–5 days. His family history is strongly positive for gout, with both brothers having had multiple attacks. He has no history of renal calculi. He is known to be hypertensive and is taking a thiazide diuretic. In the past there has been some concern about elevated creatinine levels. He has been told to avoid NSAIDs but tends to take Goody's Powders quite frequently.

Exam reveals a large African-American gentleman. Height 6'2", weight 372. He has obvious acromegalic features with extremely large hands and skull. His right 1st MTP joint is very tender and erythematous. Special investigations reveal a blood glucose of 272, creatinine of 2.1, hemoglobin of 9.8, WBC of 13.7, and platelet count of 373. His ESR is 92.

Which of the following statements apply to this patient?

A. It is most likely that he has gout. He should be given high dose ibuprofen.
B. He should be initiated on allopurinol 300 mg qd STAT.
C. He should be initiated on probenecid 500 mg bid.
D. Given the fact that he is diabetic, oral corticosteroids should be avoided. The most likely diagnosis is gout. NSAIDs are contraindicated, given his renal dysfunction. Therefore, an attempt should be made to aspirate the right 1st MTP joint, perhaps under fluoroscopy, and local corticosteroids should be injected.

443.

A 34-year-old woman presents with a 3-month history of photosensitivity, intermittent rash on her face and cheeks, and diffuse myalgias. She has bilateral arthritis of the wrists. Her physical examination today is unremarkable except for the rash on her face/cheeks.

Laboratory:
ESR 35 mm/hr
WBC 7,600/mm^3 and a normal differential
Hemoglobin 11.0 g/dL
ANA is positive
Anti-dsDNA is positive
Anti SS-A is positive
Anti-histone antibodies are positive
C3 and C4 are low

Which of the following is true regarding the laboratory findings and her history/physical examination?

A. High levels of anti-dsDNA and low complement levels are associated with increased disease activity and development of nephritis.
B. The positive anti-histone antibody indicates she has drug induced lupus.
C. Anti-Sm is positive in these patients > 75% of the time.
D. DR2 allele is associated with anti-Ro/SS-A.
E. Elevated anti-U1RNP would suggest a worse prognosis in her.

444.

A 30-year-old woman with SLE presents and reports that she is pregnant.

Which of the following is not true with regard to SLE and pregnancy?

A. She has an increased risk of spontaneous abortion.
B. If the mother has anti-histone antibodies, this results in an increased risk of complete heart block.
C. The infant will have an increased risk of thrombocytopenia.
D. There is an increased risk for neonatal lupus.
E. There is an increased risk of complete heart block in the infant.

445.

A woman presents to the ED with her 3rd spontaneous abortion.

Which of the following antibodies is associated with an increased risk of this occurring?

    A. Anti-Ro/SS-A
    B. Anti-La/SS-B
    C. c-ANCA
    D. Anticardiolipin antibody
    E. Antihistone antibody

446.

You suspect a woman with recurrent spontaneous abortions has anticardiolipin antibody.

What do you expect her coagulation studies to show?

    A. Her PTT will be normal.
    B. She will have Factor VII deficiency.
    C. Her PTT will correct when her plasma is mixed with normal.
    D. Her PTT will not correct when her plasma is mixed with normal.
    E. Anticardiolipin does not affect coagulation.

447.

A 62-year-old man with a long history of osteoarthritis of the hips and knees presents with new onset of severe pain in his right hip. The pain is so severe that he cannot roll over to sleep on his right side because of the discomfort. The pain is exacerbated by any movement of his right hip.

Physical examination is significant only for eliciting severe pain with palpation of the lateral aspect of his right hip. The pain is especially exacerbated by abduction of the hip. He has no skin lesions or lymphadenopathy.

Which of the following is the best treatment for this patient?

    A. Surgery
    B. NSAIDs
    C. Vancomycin and ceftriaxone
    D. Oral prednisone
    E. Steroid injection

448.

Which of the following therapies for rheumatoid arthritis is associated with retinopathy?

A. Methotrexate
B. Gold
C. Hydroxychloroquine
D. Penicillamine
E. Prednisone

449.

A 64-year-old woman with diabetes complains of pain in her right shoulder. The pain is worse at night. She had a pacemaker placed about 5 months ago on the right side. Additionally, she had a mastectomy 8 months ago for breast cancer. You note that she can abduct her right shoulder only to 60 degrees when you stabilize her scapula on that side. She does not have impingement. She does not have pain when supination of the forearm is resisted (Yergason test).

Which of the following is most likely, based on her history?

A. Rotator cuff tendonitis
B. Frozen shoulder (adhesive capsulitis)
C. Bicipital tendonitis
D. Subacromial bursitis
E. Rotator cuff tear

450.

A 50-year-old Caucasian woman presents with aching in her bilateral shoulder muscles and hip joints for the past month. She has tried over-the-counter medications, such as acetaminophen and ibuprofen, without relief. She has no energy and has not had any associated headaches. In the mornings she is quite stiff. She has had pain in her fingers for many years. She has noted some decline in her vision and feels weak.

On examination there is no evidence of proximal muscle weakness. She has no tenderness and no heliotropic rash is present. Her ESR is 90.

Which of the following is the most likely diagnosis?

A. Rheumatoid arthritis
B. Osteoarthritis
C. SLE
D. Polymyalgia rheumatica (PMR)
E. Ankylosing spondylitis

ALLERGY / IMMUNOLOGY

451.

A 17-year-old female comes to your office with the complaint of congestion, sinus pressure, and low-grade fever.

Physical Exam:
Her nasal turbinates are very swollen. She has post-nasal drainage and maxillary sinus tenderness.
Lungs are clear.

Past Medical History:
She has had numerous episodes of sinusitis (2 documented with CT scans).
She has milk allergy (causes diarrhea) and quite a few environmental allergies.
Frequent episodes of diarrhea.
No hospitalizations.
Immunizations are up-to-date.

You treat her for sinusitis and order which of the following test(s)?

A. Serum IgA levels
B. Neutrophil nitroblue tetrazolium dye reduction test (NBT)
C. Abdominal ultrasound
D. Calcium level
E. Serum IgE levels

452.

You are seeing a 12-month-old male in the Emergency Department who appears to have pneumococcal meningitis. He is on the appropriate therapy. On review of his past medical history, you note he has had sepsis at age 8 months (caused by *Haemophilus influenzae*), pneumonia at age 10 months, and otitis media several times in between. Mother reports he had been healthy until around 8 months of age. He was born term without complications and was breast-fed until 4 months of age. He is up-to-date on immunizations except he has had only 2 Prevnar (conjugated pneumococcal vaccine) shots due to shortage. Lab reveals normal platelet size and number. You expect an immune disorder and order the appropriate tests.

Which of the following is the most likely diagnosis?

A. X-linked agammaglobulinemia (Bruton disease)
B. No immunodeficiency
C. IgA deficiency
D. DiGeorge anomaly
E. Wiskott-Aldrich syndrome

453.

You are seeing an 11-month-old male in the emergency room for a fever that started yesterday. He has been very irritable. He has had cold symptoms but no vomiting or diarrhea. Mother is frustrated because it seems her son is "always sick." He does not attend daycare but is in the church nursery once a week. He has had multiple ear infections and pneumonia twice. He is up-to-date on his shots except Prevnar (conjugated pneumococcal vaccine) because there has been a shortage—he has received only one so far. The only other significant finding in the review of systems is he has had a dry rash for several weeks.

On physical exam, he is fussy but consolable. His right tympanic membrane is bulging, and he has nasal congestion and cervical lymphadenopathy. He has multiple dry eczematous patches on his trunk, arms, and legs. He also has petechiae on his arms and legs. Spleen tip is palpable. The remainder of the exam is normal.

You order a CBC that shows small platelets with low count, upper-end normal WBC count, and low hemoglobin and hematocrit.

Which of the following is this child's diagnosis?

    A. Wiskott-Aldrich syndrome (WAS)
    B. Another viral infection
    C. Leukemia
    D. Atopic dermatitis with superinfection
    E. Idiopathic thrombocytopenic purpura

454.

Marion Cohen is a 22-year-old who presents with severe urticaria, facial flushing, and tongue swelling after a bee sting. Her sister had a similar reaction to contrast dye.

How does a bee sting cause anaphylaxis?

    A. By causing an IgE mediated event against protein-hapten conjugants
    B. By causing a direct activation of mediator release from mast cells, basophils, or both
    C. By causing an IgE mediated reaction against the proteins in the sting media
    D. Through a deficiency of C1 esterase inhibitor
    E. By causing an IgA mediated reaction against protein-hapten conjugants

455.

A 45-year-old woman presents to the Emergency Department immediately after receiving a bee sting. She has a past history of anaphylaxis and had lost her EpiPen. She has urticaria but is not having hypotension.

Which of the following is indicated?

    A. Give epinephrine 1/1,000 0.5 cc IV
    B. Give epinephrine 1/1,000 0.5 cc SQ
    C. Give IV Solu-Medrol 2 mg/kg IV
    D. Start beta-blocker
    E. Give epinephrine 1/10,000 0.5 cc SQ

456.

A 50-year-old man was in his usual state of good health until 2 months ago when he started having problems with angioedema and laryngeal stridor. He experienced recurring episodes of swelling of his lips, tongue, and suborbital areas, which were painful but did not itch very much. He had no hives or wheezing with these episodes. His examination shows non-pitting edema of his face and 4 extremities.

Laboratory shows a normal WBC with normal differential. Electrolytes are normal. C1 esterase inhibitor serum level is very low. C1q, C2, C4, and C3 levels are also quite low.

Which of the following is the most likely diagnosis?

A. Reaction to an ACE inhibitor
B. Hereditary angioedema
C. Lymphoma
D. Allergy to foods
E. Insect hypersensitivity

457.

A 41-year-old man is working in Greece and Turkey on a movie production. He runs outdoors regularly to help keep his "star" looks. While filming, he is stung by a bee. He quickly develops anaphylaxis and requires intubation and aggressive cardiorespiratory support. He recovers well and returns to shooting the movie the next week.

Which of the following are true about anaphylactic reactions?

A. Absence of skin findings (urticaria, etc.) rules out anaphylaxis.
B. Anaphylaxis always begins within 5–10 minutes after antigen exposure.
C. Anaphylaxis is IgE mediated.
D. Anaphylactoid reactions are IgE mediated.
E. Radiocontrast dye more commonly causes anaphylaxis and not anaphylactoid reactions.

458.

A 30-year-old woman presents with a history of recurrent edema of the lips and face. She does not have urticaria with these episodes. She has come to the Emergency Department on numerous occasions thinking she has had an allergic reaction and is given epinephrine without any response. The edema gradually resolves over 1–2 days. Her brother and her father have had similar episodes but are much less affected.

What is the most likely etiology of her recurrent edema?

A. Hereditary IgE hypergammaglobulinemia
B. Decrease in C1-inhibitor
C. Terminal complement deficiency
D. Atopic dermatitis
E. Arthus hypersensitivity reaction

459.

A 20-year-old man is bitten by a rattlesnake. He is hospitalized, and equine antivenin is administered because of incipient compartment syndrome. Twelve days later he presents with swelling of his ankles, knees, and hands. He also develops fever. Urinalysis shows 3+ proteinuria.

Which of the following is the most likely cause of his symptoms?

   A. Late toxic effect of snake venom
   B. Henoch-Schönlein purpura
   C. Nephrotic syndrome
   D. Juvenile rheumatoid arthritis
   E. Serum sickness

460.

A patient with perennial allergic rhinitis is skin test positive to dust mites.

Appropriate avoidance measures for dust mites include which of the following?

   A. Encasings for bedding and HEPA air filtration for the bedroom
   B. Encasings for the bedding and frequent laundering of linens
   C. Frequent laundering of linens and HEPA air filtration
   D. Keeping windows closed
   E. None of the above

461.

A patient with perennial allergic rhinitis is skin test positive to *Alternaria*.

Which of the following interventions are reasonable for avoidance of *Alternaria*?

   A. Encasings for bedding and HEPA air filtration for the bedroom
   B. Encasings for the bedding and frequent laundering of linens
   C. Frequent laundering of linens and HEPA air filtration
   D. Keeping windows closed

462.

A 17-year-old is seen for mouth breathing and chronic rhinorrhea. His symptoms do not improve with antihistamines. He denies nasal itching or eye symptoms. He has used topical nasal steroids with poor compliance but possibly some benefit.

Which of the following is the most likely diagnosis?

A. Allergic rhinitis
B. Idiopathic rhinitis (non-allergic rhinitis)
C. Sinusitis
D. Foreign body
E. Adenoidal hypertrophy

463.

Which of the following is <u>not</u> associated with severe combined immunodeficiency (SCID)?

A. Absent T-cell and B-cell function
B. A large thymus
C. Very few circulating lymphocytes (usually)
D. No tonsils or lymph nodes usually
E. Commonly early and severe infections—viruses, bacteria, and opportunistic

464.

Which of the following is true with regards to DiGeorge syndrome?

A. DiGeorge syndrome is not associated with hypoparathyroidism.
B. Immune deficits in most with DiGeorge syndrome are minimal except for those with "complete DiGeorge."
C. Facial abnormalities do not occur.
D. Thymic abnormalities do not occur.
E. Cardiac abnormalities never occur.

465.

Which time of year are grass allergens likely to be the highest?

A. Spring
B. Summer
C. Fall
D. Winter
E. All year round

466.

Which of the following is true with regards to skin testing for allergens?

A. They have good positive predictive value for inhalants.
B. They have good positive predictive value for foods.
C. They have poor negative predictive value for foods.
D. They have poor negative predictive value for inhalants.
E. Antihistamine therapy will not suppress responses.

467.

Which of the following is an example of delayed hypersensitivity (Type IV)?

A. After tetanus immunization
B. Hives
C. Allergic rhinitis
D. Tuberculin sensitivity
E. Peanut allergy

468.

Which of the following is <u>not</u> an example of immediate hypersensitivity?

A. Peanut allergy
B. Egg allergy
C. Allergic rhinitis
D. Bee sting
E. Reaction to Td immunization

469.

Allergic reactions to which of the following are <u>not</u> IgE mediated?

A. Skin prick testing
B. Contrast dye
C. Bee sting
D. Wasp sting
E. Food allergy

470.

Which of the following statements regarding pneumonitis is true?

A. Hypersensitivity pneumonitis is cell mediated and immune complex mediated.
B. Allergic bronchopulmonary aspergillosis (ABPA) is not IgE mediated.
C. Hypersensitivity pneumonitis is IgE mediated.
D. Both allergic bronchopulmonary aspergillosis and hypersensitivity pneumonitis will respond to allergy injections.
E. Neither allergic bronchopulmonary aspergillosis nor hypersensitivity pneumonitis will respond to corticosteroids.

471.

Which of the following is <u>not</u> true about IgA deficiency?

A. Its incidence is as high as 1/600.
B. Sinopulmonary infections may be increased in these patients.
C. Recurrent giardiasis may be a problem.
D. IgA sprue can occur.
E. It is associated with Wiskott-Aldrich syndrome.

472.

Which of the following does <u>not</u> aggravate mastocytosis?

A. Cold
B. Heat
C. Alcohol
D. Aspirin
E. Cromolyn

473.

A patient has a splenectomy.

Which of the following organisms is <u>not</u> associated with an increased risk of infection?

A. *Streptococcus pneumoniae*
B. *Haemophilus influenzae*
C. *Neisseria meningitidis*
D. Rotavirus
E. Pneumococcus

474.

Which of the following should you check for in a patient with meningococcemia?

A. ANA
B. CH50
C. Factor VIII deficiency
D. IgA level
E. Anti-thymus antibodies

475.

HLA-B27 is a common antibody in some disorders.

Which of the following is <u>not</u> associated with a positive HLA-B27 level?

    A. Ankylosing spondylitis
    B. Acute anterior uveitis
    C. Reiter syndrome
    D. Psoriatic arthritis
    E. Rheumatoid arthritis

476.

A 17-year-old boy has a history of having had an anaphylactic reaction to a wasp sting 3 years ago. He presents to the ED 20 minutes after having received a wasp sting to his right shoulder.

Which of the following would <u>not</u> be considered in the treatment of this patient?

    A. IV cimetidine
    B. Solu-Medrol 125 mg IV
    C. Diphenhydramine 50 mg IV
    D. Epinephrine 1:1,000 0.2–0.5 cc IV
    E. Aminophylline 4 mg/kg IV

477.

How does contrast dye cause an anaphylactoid reaction?

    A. By causing an IgG-mediated reaction against protein-hapten conjugants
    B. By causing an IgE-mediated event against protein-hapten conjugants
    C. By causing a direct activation of mediator release from mast cells, basophils, or both
    D. Because the dye induces complement activation
    E. By causing an IgE-mediated reaction against the proteins in the dye media.

DERMATOLOGY

478.

A 33-year-old health-care worker requests smallpox vaccination. She has a history of asthma, chronic eczema, and depression.

Which of the following treatments would you recommend?

A. No vaccine because she is a health-care worker.
B. No vaccine because eczema is a contraindication.
C. No vaccine because asthma is a contraindication.
D. No vaccine because depression is a contraindication.
E. OK to vaccinate.

479.

A 37-year-old man comes in for a routine physical examination. You do a thorough examination and find only a pigmented lesion present on his left back. He states that the lesion has been present as long as he can remember—probably since he was born. The lesion does not itch or bleed. He has noted, however, that the color has changed a little and is no longer as homogeneous as it has been.

Which of the following statements is true?

A. One of the first signs of malignancy is bleeding.
B. Change in the color of the lesion warrants further workup for potential malignancy.
C. One of the first signs of malignancy is tenderness.
D. Early diagnosis of this lesion would not affect prognosis.
E. It is unlikely that the lesion, if it really has been present since birth, would be malignant.

480.

You see a 17-year-old female for a rash. She has had no fever and does not appear ill. Her mother reports that her daughter had "ringworm" on her back about a week ago, but that seems better. She woke up this morning and now has the rash on her arms, back, and stomach. On physical examination, she is alert and looks well. Her temperature is 99 degrees. She has slight nasal congestion and multiple small, oval, scaling pink papules on her trunk. You notice that these papules follow the lines of skin cleavage. Otherwise her exam is unremarkable.

You tell the mother your diagnosis, and she wants to know what treatment you recommend.

A. You refer her immediately to a dermatologist.
B. You recommend that she apply a topical anti-fungal cream three times per day.
C. She should absolutely avoid the sun.
D. You start her on a 10-day course of amoxicillin.
E. You reassure her that this is a self-limited process and that sunlight may help to accelerate remission.

481.

A 30-year-old nurse works on a general children's ward of a hospital. She develops herpes zoster in an 8th thoracic dermatome. She complains of itching but otherwise is without complaint. Her Med/Peds physician places her on valacyclovir, and she asks about returning to work.

When can she return to work?

    A. She must wait until 6 days after the appearance of the rash or until all of the lesions are crusted over.
    B. She must wait until all of the lesions are crusted over.
    C. As long as the lesion is kept covered by her clothes, she may return to work now.
    D. She can return to work after she has been on the medication for 48 hours.
    E. She can return to work in 10 days.

482.

A 28-year-old banker comes to see you because of vesicles on sun exposed areas, which have been present episodically for seven years. He has used alcohol to excess for many years. He takes no medications, and has not seen a physician for many years. Your evaluation confirms a diagnosis of porphyria cutanea tarda (PCT).

What other diagnosis should you consider?

    A. Paraneoplastic pemphigus
    B. Urinary tract infection
    C. Acanthosis nigricans
    D. Hepatitis C
    E. Hepatitis D

483.

A 19-year-old male college student presents with a diffuse maculopapular rash that is on his trunk, head, neck, palms, and soles. He also has generalized lymphadenopathy. He has a 4-week history of anal pain.

Which of the following tests is likely to identify the etiology of his rash?

    A. Skin biopsy
    B. Blood culture
    C. Penile and rectal swab sent in chocolate agar
    D. RPR
    E. Rectal swab for herpes simplex

484.

A 30-year-old man presents with a series of boils on his back. Cultures are taken and reveal methicillin-resistant *Staphylococcus aureus*. Sensitivities return, and he is changed from cefazolin to trimethoprim/sulfamethoxazole. Soon after taking his 5th dose of the new medication, he develops a generalized redness. When lateral pressure is placed on non-blistered skin, it sloughs off.

Which of the following does he most likely have?

A. Erythema multiforme
B. Lupus erythematosus
C. Dermatomyositis
D. Toxic epidermal necrolysis
E. Atopic dermatitis

485.

A very youthful 40-year-old woman is found to have seborrheic keratoses on her trunk just as her father did at her age.

Which one of the following statements is true?

A. Seborrheic keratoses may be several colors.
B. Seborrheic keratoses can sometimes become malignant.
C. Seborrheic keratoses can be markers of malignancy.
D. Seborrheic keratoses are not found on the scalp.

486.

A 55-year-old man has developed an ulceration of his leg with undermining at the periphery and a violaceous hue. After appropriate testing, no bacteria or fungus was found. He was in good general health except for severe rheumatoid arthritis.

Which of the following is the most likely diagnosis?

A. Urticaria
B. Pyoderma gangrenosum
C. Factitious ulcer
D. None of the above

487.

A 29-year-old female has flushing associated with diarrhea, wheezing and hypertension. She does not have pruritus or urticaria.

Of the systemic diseases she could have, which of the following is the most likely?

A. Mastocytosis
B. Carcinoid syndrome
C. Pheochromocytoma
D. Alcohol intoxication

488.

A 24-year-old woman was found to have erythematous scaling patches in the scalp, brows, and nasolabial fold.

Which of the following medications will <u>not</u> treat the seborrheic dermatitis of her face?

    A. Ketoconazole cream
    B. Penciclovir cream
    C. Ciclopirox gel
    D. Low potency topical steroid

489.

An HIV-positive gentleman was found to have genital warts. He does not like pain and refuses cryotherapy.

Which of the following is the most effective therapy that will <u>not</u> cause painful lesions?

    A. Cantharone
    B. Podophyllin
    C. Trichloroacetic acid
    D. Imiquimod cream

490.

A 15-year-old boy comes in with a rash on his trunk. He is a Caucasian male with dark crusty lesions on his back and chest. They seem to become darker when exposed to sunlight. You do a scraping of one of the lesions, and the results are presented in Figure 4 (see photo at back of book).

Which of the following organisms is responsible for his lesions?

    A. *Tinea capitis*
    B. *Malassezia furfur (Pityrosporon orbiculare)*
    C. *Candida albicans*
    D. *Candida marneffei*
    E. *Cryptococcus neoformans*

491.

Which virus is responsible for the findings in Figure 5 (see photo at back of book)?

    A. Herpes simplex type I
    B. Herpes simplex type II
    C. Varicella virus
    D. Cytomegalovirus
    E. It could be either A or B

492.

A 22-year-old woman presents with hundreds of 2–5 mm scaly red papules on the trunk and extremities that are moderately pruritic. The lesions appeared abruptly approximately 2 weeks prior to examination and quickly spread. Upon further questioning, the patient reported having a sore throat the prior month.

Which of the following is the most likely diagnosis for this patient?

    A. Guttate psoriasis
    B. Erythema multiforme
    C. Pityriasis rosea
    D. Secondary syphilis
    E. Contact dermatitis

493.

An 18-year-old male presents with many closed and open comedones involving the face, chest, and back. In addition, he has approximately 30 to 40 inflammatory papules and pustules.

Which of the following would be an appropriate treatment for this patient?

    A. Topical benzoyl peroxide.
    B. Topical retinoid therapy.
    C. Combination topical benzoyl peroxide and topical antibiotic.
    D. Oral antibiotic therapy with doxycycline.
    E. All of the choices could be appropriate.

OB / GYN

494.

A 27-year-old woman G1P0 presents with nausea, vomiting, abdominal pain and jaundice. She is 33 weeks pregnant. Labs: AST 333, ALT 269, Bili 7.9, WBC 13,700, PLT 159,000, HCT 34

Which of the following is the most likely diagnosis?

A. Hyperemesis gravidarum
B. HELLP syndrome
C. Primary biliary cirrhosis
D. Acute fatty liver of pregnancy
E. Alcoholic hepatitis

495.

A 25-year-old Cambodian woman is seen for primary care. She has not received any previous vaccinations except for one dose of tetanus vaccine 1 year ago. She is 3 months pregnant.

What do you recommend as additional treatment?

A. Complete the tetanus series
B. Tetanus + MMR
C. Tetanus + MMR + oral polio vaccine
D. No immunizations

496.

The EDC (expected date of confinement) may be calculated by using various methods.

Which of the following statements is not true?

A. In a woman with 28-day cycles, 280 days after the onset of the last menstrual period determines the EDC.
B. That little wheel thingee can be used.
C. Subtracting 3 months from the first day of the last menses and then adding 7 days will give you the month and day; finally, increasing the year by 1 determines the EDC.
D. In women who use steroidal contraceptives immediately before pregnancy, the EDC is easily calculated.
E. In women with irregular menses, calculating the EDC is less precise.

497.

A 25-year-old woman whom you've been following for the past 4 years for ulcerative colitis comes to the office with the joyful news that she and her husband are expecting their first child. She's 8 weeks pregnant at this time. She has had ulcerative colitis since the age of 20. A past colonoscopy has demonstrated this is distal disease or proctosigmoiditis. She has had approximately 2 or 3 flares of disease activity each year, each time being manifest as frequent bloody stools with mucus and tenesmus. During those times she has responded to oral prednisone added to her regimen of mesalamine. Previously she was on 1.6 g/day of mesalamine. Over the past 6 months, this was increased to 3.2 gm of mesalamine/day, and this is seen to benefit her with fewer flares of the colitis.

Her past medical history is otherwise unremarkable. Review of systems is negative for joint pain, skin lesions, mouth lesions, or painful eye lesions.

Physical exam is normal.

For this outpatient with ulcerative colitis and new pregnancy, which of the following would be the most appropriate treatment?

A. Continue mesalamine in its current dose
B. Discontinue the mesalamine and initiate low dose prednisone 10 mg/day
C. Add azathioprine to the mesalamine with the hopes of preventing any flares during pregnancy
D. Continue mesalamine in the same dose and add 20 mg prednisone/day
E. Schedule colonoscopy to determine the disease activity prior to any changes in therapy.

498.

A 40-year-old pregnant woman presents for evaluation. She is 28 weeks by dates and has been doing well. Today she awoke with burning on urination, and you have determined that she has a UTI and have sent a urine culture to confirm. She is allergic to penicillin (rash).

Which of the following agents can you <u>not</u> use in this woman for treatment of her UTI?

A. Gentamicin
B. Trimethoprim/sulfamethoxazole
C. Ceftriaxone
D. Ciprofloxacin
E. Azactam

499.

A 25-year-old pregnant woman has a history of mild hypertension, treated with hydrochlorothiazide (HCTZ). When her pregnancy was diagnosed, her obstetrician discontinued the HCTZ and has been watching her blood pressure. She is now 20 weeks pregnant and her blood pressure is 140/100. Urinalysis is normal.

Which of the following would be the most appropriate recommendation?

A. Start alpha-methyldopa 250 mg bid
B. Resume the HCTZ at 12.5 mg/day
C. Start enalapril 10 mg/day
D. Start verapamil 80 mg bid

500.

A young woman with diabetes whom you have been following presents and asks about pregnancy. She wants to know what her optimal therapy should be.

Which of the following would you recommend?

A. Her glycosylated hemoglobin should be targeted for 6.0 before and during pregnancy.
B. Her glycosylated hemoglobin should be targeted for 6.0 during pregnancy.
C. Her glycosylated hemoglobin should be targeted for 7.0 during pregnancy.
D. Her glycosylated hemoglobin should be targeted for 7.0 before and during pregnancy.
E. She needs to be off insulin completely before she can become pregnant.

501.

What is the most common reason for postcoital bleeding in a young woman, assuming that Pap smears have been negative and she has no other symptoms?

A. Cervical cancer
B. Nabothian cyst
C. Cervical HSV
D. Cervical syphilis
E. Endocervical polyp

502.

A 31-year-old pregnant woman (20 weeks) presents for evaluation. She is found to have a positive urine culture with > 100,000 colonies of *E. coli*. She is completely asymptomatic.

Which of the following would you recommend?

A. Treat with ciprofloxacin
B. Treat with doxycycline
C. Treat with amoxicillin
D. Treat with clindamycin
E. No treatment is necessary

503.

An elderly woman is being evaluated for urinary incontinence. She has had a 10-year history of incontinence that occurs when she laughs or sneezes. Recently, however, this has changed, and it occurs when she stands up from a chair. A urinalysis is normal.

Which of the following is the likely diagnosis?

A. Bladder spasms
B. Stress incontinence
C. Neurologic deterioration
D. Multiple sclerosis
E. Pituitary tumor

504.

A pregnant woman presents with a newly positive RPR. She is allergic to penicillin (she has anaphylaxis).

Which of the following do you recommend now?

- A. Begin doxycycline for 28 days
- B. Begin imipenem x 7 days
- C. Desensitize her and treat with penicillin
- D. Give her ceftriaxone in the ICU
- E. Wait till she delivers and then treat her with doxycycline for 28 days; the baby can then be safely treated with penicillin

OPHTHALMOLOGY

505.

A 15-year-old male presents to your clinic with the complaint of right eye trauma. He was playing basketball and was hit in the eye with an elbow. He says he can see OK. On physical exam, his right eyelid is slightly swollen. The orbital bone feels intact. Extraocular muscles are intact. There is blood filling approximately 15% of the anterior chamber.

Which of the following is <u>not</u> appropriate treatment?

A. Non-steroidal antiinflammatory medication
B. Bed rest
C. Cycloplegic eyedrops (atropine)
D. Corticosteroid eyedrops
E. Protective shield

506.

A 28-year-old is being evaluated for anisocoria. Her left pupil is small and round compared with the right pupil in room light. When you place her in a darkened room, this difference is increased. The left pupil responds briskly to light, constricts with pilocarpine administration, and dilates with atropine. Minimal dilatation is produced by 4% cocaine.

Which of the following indicates where her lesion is located?

A. Left sympathetic chain
B. Left optic nerve
C. Left iris
D. Left third nerve
E. Right occipital lobe

507.

A 70-year-old man presents with sudden vision loss. He has no pain, and on physical examination of the eye you note a cherry red spot.

Which of the following is the most likely diagnosis?

A. Tay-Sachs disease
B. Retinal artery occlusion
C. Retinal detachment
D. Endophthalmitis
E. Occipital cortex infarct

508.

An 18-year-old woman comes to your office complaining of a unilateral throbbing headache that was preceded by "seeing flashing lights." The headache worsened over a 30-minute period, has been present for four hours, and seems to be getting better. The headache is severe. She says that she was nauseous with the headache and vomited several times. The headache is exacerbated by loud noises. Her physical examination is normal, and in particular, she has no weakness or numbness. There is no papilledema on funduscopic examination. Serum tests are normal.

What is the most likely diagnosis?

- A. Pseudotumor cerebri
- B. Cluster headache
- C. Migraine headache
- D. Tension headache
- E. Subarachnoid hemorrhage

509.

A 60-year-old man comes in for routine checkup. He notes that his vision has gradually gotten worse, especially in the right eye. See Figure 6 (back of book).

With which of the following is his eye exam (Figure 6) most consistent?

- A. Cataract
- B. CMV retinitis
- C. Hypertensive retinopathy
- D. Glaucoma
- E. Macular degeneration

510.

An 18-year-old college student presents with floaters and blurry vision. She is HIV positive and has a CD4 count of 20.

What etiology are you most concerned about in this young woman?

- A. Toxoplasmosis
- B. Cytomegalovirus
- C. *Cryptococcus*
- D. Coccidioidomycosis
- E. HIV retinopathy

511.

An 18-year-old woman presents for routine checkup. She is without complaint and has not noted any visual disturbances. She is HIV positive and has a CD4 count of 520. On funduscopic examination you note cotton wool spots without hemorrhage.

What is the most likely etiology for her eye findings?

    A. Toxoplasmosis
    B. Cytomegalovirus
    C. *Cryptococcus*
    D. Coccidioidomycosis
    E. HIV retinopathy

512.

Ken B. is a 45-year-old man with worsening vision for the past few months. He is a proofreader for a major publishing company in Colorado.

What is the most likely etiology for his vision changes?

    A. Optic neuritis
    B. Acute angle glaucoma
    C. Retinal hemorrhage
    D. Presbyopia
    E. Macular degeneration

513.

A 50-year-old man with no health problems presents with vision loss. You note that it mainly is at the periphery on visual field testing. It is bilateral peripheral vision loss.

What is a possible explanation for this bilateral vision loss?

    A. Open-angle glaucoma
    B. Closed-angle glaucoma
    C. Optic chiasm mass
    D. Multiple sclerosis
    E. Occipital tumor

PSYCHIATRY

514.

A 30-year-old woman presents with symptoms of depression. She has successfully been treated for depression in the past but gained 20 lbs. on therapy, and she is reluctant to take medications because of fear of weight gain.

What antidepressant would be the best option for her in regard to weight gain?

- A. Amitriptyline
- B. Paroxetine
- C. Mirtazapine
- D. Venlafaxine

515.

A 16-year-old girl is brought in by her parents. She meets with you privately, and you discuss what is going on in her life. She relates that she has been really tired lately. She says she no longer has interest in school or her friends and that she can't sleep. When asked about school she says that she is a poor student, although she tells you that last quarter she made all As and Bs. She reports that she misses meals frequently because of lack of appetite. The patient notes that everyone around her seems to irritate her. Additionally, last week she started having abdominal pain that kept her out of school for 3 days. The pain does not awaken her at night and starts after she awakens in the morning. She complains of intermittent constipation, has noticed that she cannot fall asleep some nights, and that most mornings she would rather stay in bed than get up.

Her physical examination is essentially normal except for mildly pale conjunctiva. Otherwise her abdominal, developmental, and neurological examinations reveal no abnormalities. She is at Tanner Stage IV.

What diagnosis would you put at the top of your list?

- A. Depression
- B. Hypothyroidism
- C. Hyperthyroidism
- D. Vitamin deficiency
- E. Oppositional behavior

516.

A 40-year-old man presents with a history of bipolar disorder. He is taking lithium and now has developed ataxia and incoordination. He started on a new medication last week.

Which of the following is true about lithium toxicity and/or its metabolism?

- A. Tinnitus is uncommon in toxicity.
- B. ACE inhibitors can decrease excretion of lithium.
- C. Thiazides increase excretion of lithium.
- D. Anuria is more likely than polyuria in cases of toxicity.
- E. Constipation is more likely than diarrhea in cases of toxicity.

517.

A 16-year-old girl is brought to you for evaluation of nocturnal enuresis. Several appointments have been missed over the past year. Her father, a professor at a nearby college, is very concerned to the point of demanding an immediate solution. The girl was dry between the ages of 5 and 14, but over the past two years has had frequent episodes of bed-wetting. Her school performance has also declined, and she rarely leaves her room. The father confides that there has been domestic discord between him and his spouse for the last year. The father insists on being present during the physical exam, where nothing abnormal is found. The patient's blood pressure and vital signs are unremarkable. She is Tanner stage IV, and has a normal neurologic exam.

Which of the following would be the most appropriate next step in evaluation?

A. Obtain electrolytes, creatinine clearance, and an IVP
B. Begin a program of bed-wetting alarms and bladder training exercises
C. Begin a trial of desmopressin (DDAVP®)
D. Have a private conversation with the patient about possible abuse
E. Reassure the patient and ask her to return for follow-up in one year

518.

An 80-year-old woman has been having gradually worsening short-term memory for 3 years. On neurological exam, she is pleasant but has difficulty naming objects such as a stethoscope. She has trouble following complex commands. There is no focal weakness or numbness. There has been no incontinence, and her gait is slow, but normal. There is no resting tremor, masked facies, or festinating gait.

Which of the following is the most likely diagnosis?

A. Pick dementia
B. Alzheimer dementia
C. Creutzfeldt-Jacob disease
D. Herpes encephalitis
E. Stroke

519.

A 65-year-old man with dementia of the Alzheimer's type has become increasingly agitated and aggressive over the past 2 weeks. He lives at home, and his wife fears for his safety as well as her own.

Which of the following is most appropriate initial pharmacologic management?

A. Lorazepam 0.5 mg tid
B. Haloperidol 1 mg daily
C. Carbamazepine 100 mg tid
D. Trazodone 50 mg tid
E. Phenytoin 100 mg tid

520.

Two days after surgical repair of a broken arm, an 80-year-old woman thinks she is in Nebraska (she lives in Florida) and that the nurses are trying to hurt her. She is being physically restrained. Before hospitalization she lived alone in Fort Meyers, Florida. Although she is increasingly frail and forgetful, no new problems were identified on preoperative evaluation. She sleeps deeply, and on arousal from sleep, she is disoriented and drowsy. Mental status testing shows perseveration and visual hallucinations.

Which of the following is the most likely diagnosis?

   A. Schizophrenia
   B. Seizure disorder
   C. Major depressive disorder
   D. Dementia
   E. Delirium

521.

A nurse from an assisted living residence calls you about a patient of yours. Mrs. Barks is a 75-year-old woman who has a history of dementia, hypertension, and diabetes mellitus. The nurse says that Mrs. Barks has been more agitated and confused in the past few days. Mrs. Barks has been verbally and physically abusive to caretakers. Her current medications include glyburide, furosemide, and enalapril.

Which of the following is the most appropriate in the evaluation and management of this patient?

   A. Assess the patient for an acute medical problem
   B. Perform an MRI
   C. Give her lorazepam 0.5 mg x 1 and see how she reacts
   D. Give her haloperidol 0.5 mg x 1 and see how she reacts
   E. Start a trial of an SSRI antidepressant for probable depression

522.

A 65-year-old man is brought in by his son because he seems depressed. The son says that his dad is not sad or tearful, but he seems apathetic and disinterested in his usual activities. He has had difficulty thinking and concentrating and has no energy to do anything enjoyable. He has had no changes in sleep or appetite. The patient denies feelings of worthlessness or suicidal thoughts. He has not been tearful and does not complain himself of loss of energy. His physical examination shows a heart rate of 65, and his reflexes are slightly slowed. You give him a battery of tests, and his depression rating score is 20/30 on the geriatric depression rating scale.

What other test would you like to get before you begin therapy?

   A. RPR
   B. TSH
   C. CT of the head
   D. MRI of the head
   E. None, he has depression

523.

An 85-year-old man presents with his son. The son says that his dad has had increasing difficulty with driving and recently had a wreck where he ran a stop sign. Recently he says that Dad has gotten lost in the mall. His father gets angry and says that he is not having any problems.

Which of the following is the most appropriate intervention?

    A. Notify the state bureau of motor vehicles
    B. Arrange for him to take a driver's test with road testing
    C. Evaluate his cognitive status
    D. Suggest that the family hide his car keys
    E. Recommend that he not drive

524.

All of the following are true about the drug lithium <u>except</u>:

    A. It is the drug of choice for major depressive syndromes.
    B. It has many drug-drug interactions.
    C. It can be very effective therapy for bipolar-affective disorders.
    D. Toxicity manifests as depression of mental status.
    E. Hypothyroidism is a potential side effect of the drug.

525.

Which of the following are predictors of a <u>poor</u> prognosis for a patient with newly diagnosed schizophrenia?

    A. Early onset
    B. No family history of schizophrenia
    C. Good support system
    D. Precipitating factors
    E. Good premorbid functioning

526.

A patient with newly diagnosed schizophrenia is placed on therapy and is doing well. Her husband calls saying that now she has muscle spasms, tongue protrusion with twisting, and she can't keep from deviating her head and eyes to the right.

Which of the following is the likely diagnosis?

    A. Acute schizophrenia relapse
    B. Petit-mal seizures
    C. Allergic reaction
    D. Acute dystonic reaction
    E. Hyperthermic syndrome

527.

A patient with newly diagnosed schizophrenia is placed on haloperidol and is doing well. His wife calls saying that now he has muscle spasms, tongue protrusion with twisting, and he can't keep from deviating his head and eyes to the right.

Which of the following is the best initial treatment for this condition?

A. Acetaminophen
B. Aspirin
C. Propanol
D. Cool tepid baths
E. Diphenhydramine or benztropine immediately

528.

Brad Bit comes to you and says that he is very depressed. His girlfriend Jennifer has broken up with him, and he says he cannot bear to live any longer. He says that he has a plan to kill himself and that he plans to carry it out unless his girlfriend comes back to him. He is tearful and says that he needs you to give him something to calm his nerves or otherwise he will commit suicide.

Based on this history, what do you do at this point?

A. Keep him at your office for 3–4 hours, sedate him, and see if he improves over time
B. Arrange for immediate outpatient follow-up tomorrow morning
C. Arrange for a visiting nurse to check in on him tonight and tomorrow
D. Voluntary hospitalization; if he refuses, arrange appropriate follow-up tomorrow
E. Voluntary hospitalization; if he refuses, institute involuntary commitment

529.

Which of the following is true with regard to suicide in the United States?

A. People younger than 30 are at greater risk than those over 45 years of age.
B. Men attempt suicide more often than women.
C. Women are more successful in committing suicide than men.
D. The best predictor of future suicide is a past attempt.
E. All of the statements are true.

530.

The plaques that cause Alzheimer's are made up of which of the following?

A. IgA
B. IgM
C. β-amyloid protein
D. Fibrillar actin particles
E. Cholesterol

531.

What is anhedonia?

A. Inability to understand Board questions
B. Anxiety
C. Insomnia
D. Loss of pleasure from activities that usually bring pleasure
E. Hyper-alertness

532.

Which of the following are associated with Wernicke aphasia?

A. It is associated with a lesion in the posterior temporal gyrus of the dominant hemisphere.
B. You will see a right superior quadrantanopia.
C. Poor repetition.
D. Fluent speech output.
E. All of the choices are correct.

533.

A 20-year-old man from England presents with new onset of dementia, ataxia, and lethargy. You suspect "mad cow disease."

If it is mad cow disease, what type of infectious etiology is responsible?

A. A spirochete
B. A bacteria
C. A virus
D. A prion
E. A toxin

MISCELLANEOUS

534.

An 85-year-old man is brought to the ED for evaluation of weakness and nausea. He was diagnosed 10 days ago with prostatitis. His other problems include hypertension, CHF, and CRI. Meds: Carvedilol, furosemide, TMP/Sulfa, verapamil, digoxin.

Exam:
BP 100/60, P 100, T 36.9° C
Heart: Grade 2/6 SEM lower; extremity edema present

Lab: Na 132, K 6.8, BUN 37, Cr 2.3.

Which of the following is the most likely cause of his hyperkalemia?

   A. Chronic renal insufficiency
   B. Carvedilol
   C. TMP/Sulfa
   D. Verapamil
   E. Digoxin

535.

A 57-year-old woman develops watery diarrhea while in the hospital. She was treated with ceftriaxone and clindamycin for a severe foot infection. She is afebrile without abdominal pain. Stool studies show positive *C. difficile* antigen and toxin B.

Which of the following do you recommend for treatment?

   A. No treatment
   B. IV metronidazole
   C. Oral metronidazole
   D. IV vancomycin
   E. Oral vancomycin

536.

A 47-year-old woman with Type 2 DM is evaluated for hyperlipidemia. She has been treated with simvastatin for the past 8 months. Her most recent lipid panel: TC 258, HDL 39, Tri 330, LDL 154.

Which of the following changes would <u>most</u> increase the risk of toxicity?

   A. Increase simvastatin from 20 mg to 40 mg
   B. Add cholestyramine
   C. Add gemfibrozil
   D. Switch to atorvastatin 40 mg a day

537.

A 39-year-old man with a history of alcoholism presents with nausea, vomiting, ataxia, and confusion. Physical Exam: BP 80/80, Pulse 120, RR 24, neuro exam—oriented only to person.

Lab: Na 133, Glu 80, K 5.0, Cl 96, HCO_3 10, Bun 14, Cr 1.5, serum osmolality 295

Of the following, what is the most likely diagnosis?

- A. Lactic acidosis
- B. Isopropyl alcohol ingestion
- C. Salicylate ingestion
- D. Ethylene glycol ingestion
- E. Renal tubular acidosis

538.

A study is done to test a new treatment for heart failure. Patients received usual CHF treatment plus drug or usual treatment plus placebo. 10/50 patients who received the drug died and 20/50 patients who received placebo died.

What is the number needed to treat (NNT) for this new drug?

- A. 2
- B. 5
- C. 10
- D. 15
- E. 50

539.

Which of the following is <u>not</u> true?

- A. Increased prevalence increases the positive predictive value of a diagnostic test.
- B. Neither sensitivity nor specificity takes into account prevalence of the disease.
- C. Sensitivity takes into account only those who have the disease.
- D. As disease prevalence decreases, the ratio of false positives to false negatives decreases.
- E. Increasing the threshold for normal in a test will decrease the sensitivity and increase the specificity.

540.

A 19-year-old man presents to the ED tearful and agitated. He reports he took a bottle of extra strength Tylenol 4 hours ago in a suicide attempt. His physical exam is normal.
Laboratory: hemoglobin is 15.5 mg/dL; WBC 8,500
Acetaminophen level 300 mg/mL

Which of the following is the appropriate management at this point?

A. Gastric lavage
B. N-acetylcysteine
C. N-acetylcysteine + gastric lavage followed by activated charcoal
D. N-acetylcysteine + activated charcoal
E. Deferoxamine

541.

You are the physician in charge of laboratory services for your group practice. There are 3 different companies that make rapid screening tests for group A streptococcus. You need to review the performance of each test and decide which you will purchase for the coming year. Assume all culture negative patients do not have group A streptococcus infection.

Company XYZ
The rapid screening test was performed on 100 patients with culture positive group A streptococcus and 100 patients without group A streptococcus (culture negative). 95 of the culture positive patients have a positive rapid screen, and 92 of the culture negative patients have a negative test result.

The sensitivity of Company XYZ's test is:

A. 99%
B. 95%
C. 92%
D. 48%
E. 90%

542.

A 70-year-old patient and long-time friend of yours comes to the office for routine check-up. Near the end of the visit, she asks you to write a "medical condition" letter so she can get a refund on the airline ticket she purchased several months ago. She discloses that they recently lowered their fares for her flight next week, and she would like to get her money back and buy a new ticket at the lower price.

Which of the following will you decide to do?

A. Not write the letter and tell her why you cannot
B. Write a letter to the airline asking them to change their refund policy
C. Write the letter as she asks, but only this once
D. Not write the letter and report her to the airline for attempted fraud
E. Tell her to write the letter and use your name

543.

You are the physician in charge of laboratory services for your group practice. There are 3 different companies that make rapid screening tests for group A streptococcus. You need to review the performance of each test and decide which you will purchase for the coming year. Assume all culture negative patients do not have group A streptococcus infection.

Company LMR
The rapid screening test was performed on 500 patients, 200 with culture positive group A streptococcus and 300 patients without group A streptococcus (culture negative). 194 of the culture positive patients have a positive rapid screen, and 27 of the culture negative patients have a positive test result.

The specificity of Company LMR's test is:

A. 97.8%
B. 97%
C. 91%
D. 90%
E. 87.8%

544.

A 45-year-old woman presents with diarrhea for several months. She has recently noted that her stools "float" and are quite smelly in character. A Sudan stain is positive. Quantitative fecal fat studies show > 16 grams/day.

What test can you now order to potentially "rule-out" small bowel disease as a cause of malabsorption in this woman?

A. D-xylose test
B. String test
C. Ultrasound of abdomen
D. Upper GI
E. Specific antigen test of a parasite

545.

A study is designed to test a new treatment for advanced prostate cancer. Patients received usual prostate therapy plus experimental drug X, or usual treatment plus a placebo.

40/100 patients who received the drug died and 50/100 patients who received placebo died.

What is the number needed to treat (NNT) for this new drug?

A. 4
B. 5
C. 10
D. 15
E. 50

546.

You get a call from the ED physician who is examining Joe, a 16-year-old African-American who was brought by ambulance from football practice, where he collapsed after 30 minutes of exercises. He tells you that Joe had been in his normal state of good health until he collapsed and is now complaining that he hurts all over. ROS is negative for fever, vomiting, diarrhea, cold symptoms. He is on no medications.

On physical exam: T 100.2° F, HR 110, RR 25

General:	Uncomfortable due to body aches
HEENT:	WNL
Heart:	No murmur
Lungs:	CTA
Abdomen:	No masses
Extremities:	Starting to get a few petechiae on arms

Lab:
Na 131, K 6.8
Ca 6.9 (Low)
CPK 80,000 IU/L (nl 0–200)
Creatinine 2.1
Urine is brown and shows large blood with only 0–2 RBCs.
He is known to be sickle trait positive.

You tell the ED physician to:

A. Admit this patient to the floor
B. Have this patient follow up with you in clinic the next day
C. Admit the patient to the ICU and that he likely has acute rhabdomyolysis
D. Admit the patient to the ICU and that he likely has TTP
E. Admit the patient to the ICU and that he likely has sickle cell crisis

547.

A 25-year-old woman presents after an MVA. She is bleeding profusely from a left thigh injury. She is found to have a hematocrit of 19%. She is given IV fluids and is typed and crossed for transfusion. She refuses blood transfusion based on religious reasons. Her husband is with her and concurs. She continues to ooze as the vascular surgeon arrives to take her to the operating room.

Which of the following should you do?

A. Get a stat Ethics Committee consult
B. Do not give blood products
C. Get a court to rule she must receive blood
D. Give blood and get the court ruling later
E. Give blood because this is a life-threatening emergency

548.

A 40-year-old woman with end-stage breast cancer presents to you for evaluation. She has made her wishes known that she does not want mechanical ventilation. Her husband disagrees with her vehemently and says that if she becomes that ill, he will not allow the doctors to withhold therapy. She has signed a living will, and you have documented her wishes in the chart.

A month later she presents to the Emergency Department in respiratory distress and is comatose. Her husband demands that mechanical ventilation be instituted if she needs it. You determine that she does indeed require mechanical ventilation if she is to survive.

Which of the following is your next course of action?

    A. Intubate and place on mechanical ventilation at the husband's request, since she cannot give her current thoughts on this
    B. Follow her living will instructions and do not institute mechanical ventilation
    C. Get an Ethics consult
    D. Call a colleague and get her opinion
    E. Have the administrator on call make the decision

549.

A 40-year-old man presents with metastatic carcinoma of the brain, lung, and liver. His prognosis is poor, and you have no therapy to offer him. He is estranged from his wife and has made his eldest son, who is 20, his power of attorney for medical as well as legal matters.

He presents to the ED in respiratory distress and requires intubation. He is too disoriented to answer the questions you ask. His wife is present and says that she wants him intubated. His eldest son is present and says that his father had specifically requested that he not be intubated.

Which of the following is your next course of action?

    A. Intubate the patient
    B. Do not intubate the patient but make him comfortable
    C. Get an Ethics consult
    D. Get the courts to rule who should decide
    E. Ask the administrator on call

550.

A 60-year-old woman presents for routine physical examination. She has not had a physician exam in more than 15 years.

Appropriate preventative care for her now would include which of the following?

    A. Complete history and physical, Td immunization, breast examination, mammogram, Pap smear, and flexible sigmoidoscopy or colonoscopy
    B. Complete history and physical, Td immunization, breast examination, mammogram, and Pap smear
    C. Complete history and physical, breast examination, mammogram, and CBC
    D. Complete history and physical, mammogram, CBC, and flexible sigmoidoscopy or colonoscopy
    E. Complete history and physical, breast examination, mammogram, and flexible sigmoidoscopy

551.

A 16-year-old high school student recently developed acne and was prescribed an oral antibiotic. He presents now with a sudden onset of pain with swallowing anything, either liquid or solid. This has been present since yesterday. His physical exam is normal.

Which of the following would you recommend?

A. EGD
B. Trial of proton pump inhibitor
C. Hyoscyamine po before meals
D. Upper GI, x-ray, and HIV assay
E. Supportive care

552.

A pregnant 22-year-old presents at 25 weeks by dates and has been doing well. She asks if she did need medications during the pregnancy would she have them available or would she have to forgo treatment to protect her unborn child.

Which of the following agents can you use safely during pregnancy?

A. Doxycycline
B. Rifampin
C. Fosinopril
D. Ciprofloxacin
E. Erythromycin

553.

Which of the following has been shown to increase the risk of ADHD?

A. Sugar
B. Artificial flavorings
C. Salicylates
D. Fetal exposure to alcohol
E. Studying Board Review questions for 8 hours a day

554.

A 17-year-old presents and has not received any immunizations and has never had chickenpox.

Which of the following vaccines should she receive today?

A. Tdap, rotavirus vaccine
B. DT, conjugated pneumococcal, hepatitis B
C. Tdap, hepatitis B, MMR, IPV, varicella, meningococcal conjugate vaccine, hepatitis A, HPV
D. DTaP, conjugated pneumococcal, Hib, varicella, MMR
E. DTaP, conjugated pneumococcal, hepatitis B, MMR, *Haemophilus influenzae*

555.

A surgery intern cuts himself in the OR with a scalpel while sewing up a patient after surgery.

Which of the following is correct?

A. He needs a Tdap if it has been less than 5 years since his last tetanus immunization.
B. He needs a Tdap if it has been less than 10 years since his last tetanus immunization.
C. He needs a DTaP if it has been less than 10 years since his last tetanus immunization.
D. He needs a DTaP if it has been more than 10 years since his last tetanus immunization.
E. He needs a Tdap if it has been more than 10 years since his last tetanus immunization.

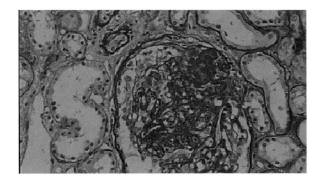

Figure 1, Nephrology, Question 242

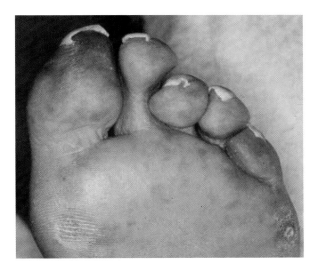

Figure 2, Nephrology, Question 243

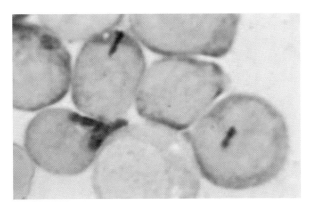

Figure 3, Hematology, Question 347

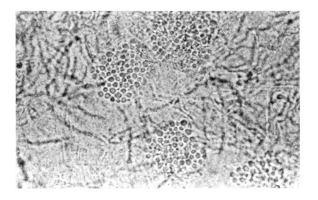

Figure 4, Dermatology, Question 490

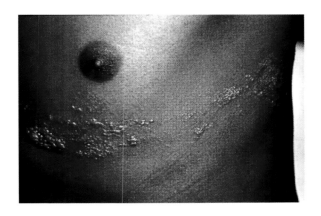

Figure 5, Dermatology, Question 491

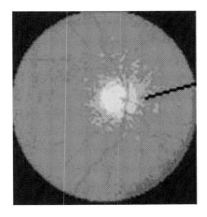

Figure 6, Ophthalmology, Question 509